1.50

Everybody Loves
THE I LOVE N

"Readers have noth   *iews*

"Its solid nutritional   om-
mend."   *ers Weekly*

"It's not only foolproof

—Dr. Nicholas Pace,
Assistant Professor
New York University School of Medicine

"*The I Love New York Diet* is a balanced, low-calorie diet
limited in fat and far superior to the fad diets so popular
in our society."

—Daniel W. Foster, M.D.
Professor of Internal Medicine
University of Texas Health Science Center, Dallas

"*The I Love New York Diet* can keep you thin in any of
the 50 states."   —Howard Cosell

"At last there's a diet that's not boring—and that you can
follow wherever you live."   —Dick Clark

"I've tried all the popular diets because, in a speaking
career that covers more than 100 banquets a year, I'm
tempted by every culinary excess known to a chef. This
book is for me!"   —Art Linkletter

"I stick to a sensible diet and together with my exercises
every day, I stay slim. I love *The I Love New York Diet*."

—Suzy Chaffee

"Bess Myerson and Bill Adler have given us a diet that
will allow people to lose weight in an easy, sensible and
responsible manner."

—Dr. Herbert Benson
Associate Professor of Medicine at
Harvard Medical School
and Director of the Division
of Behavioral Medicine
at Boston's Beth Israel Hospital

"It's a safe, simple, start-anytime, do-it-anywhere diet that anybody can follow successfully."
                    —Francine Prince
                    Author of Francine Prince's
                    New Gourmet Recipes For Dieters and Diet For Life

"Bess Myerson and Bill Adler have come up with a diet that really works and has helped people like me remain thin."
                    —Irving Mansfield

"All the attractive New Yorkers I know follow *The I Love New York Diet.*"   —Lyn Revson

"*The I Love New York Diet* not only works for New Yorkers but former New Yorkers like me who have strayed to the wilds of Washington."   —Larry King

"This highly readable, medically sound book is the Declaration of Independence for Fat People!" —Barry Farber

"My doctor put me on a diet based on the guidelines of *The I Love New York Diet* and I lost 20 pounds. It works!"
                    —Ron Nessen

The
I ♥ NY
DIET

by Bess Myerson and Bill Adler

With a foreword by Dr. Myron Winick,
Director, Institute of Human Nutrition,
Columbia University

WARNER BOOKS

A Warner Communications Company

A NOTE OF CAUTION: Though the authors and publisher of this book believe in the safety and sanity of the I Love New York Diet, and though we have been guided by responsible leaders in the health professions, we are not licensed to give medical advice. We are not doctors. Any diet must be approached with personal caution, and any wise dieter must seek the close guidance of his or her own doctor before entering any diet or exercise program. The authors and publisher specifically disclaim any liability, loss, or risk, personal or otherwise, resulting as a consequence, directly or indirectly, from the use and application of any of the contents of this book.

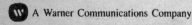

To everyone who ever stepped on a scale and winced, or looked in a mirror and wanted to hide—a diet to help you feel and look better, and the increased confidence to reach out for the fullness of life that the overfullness of our own frames too often makes difficult.

ACKNOWLEDGMENT

*We would like to thank Harold Prince
for his inestimable help
in the preparation of this book.*

Foreword

BORN IN NEW YORK, raised on its pavements and in its parks, educated in its school and universities, trained in its hospitals, I love New York. It is a city always in the center of what is important in the world, a city whose contributions to science have been as great as its contributions to music, art, and literature. It should therefore come as no surprise that more than twenty-five years ago, before the "trendy," unscientific fad diets from Scarsdale or Beverly Hills were in vogue, the Bureau of Nutrition, New York City Department of Health, developed a diet based on solid scientific data that was medically sound and reasonably easy to follow. Under the direction of Dr. Norman Jolliffe, a pioneer in modern nutrition, this diet was tested by a team of scientists on many volunteers before it was made available to the public.

In reality, this is more than a weight reduction diet; it is a pattern of eating which is designed not only to produce leanness, but also to lower the risk of heart disease and high blood pressure. When one considers when it was developed, true to its tradition, New York was far ahead of the times. This diet, which the authors choose to call the I Love New York Diet, is low in calories (the only way to produce sustained weight loss) and of a high nutrient density (the amounts of vitamins and minerals per calorie are very high). Thus the foods which are carefully chosen supply adequate amounts of all nutrients. This is in sharp contrast to those diets that promote one food (grapefruit or alcohol, for example) or one type of food (as in the Beverly Hills diet) which may be deficient in one or more important nutrients.

In addition, this diet is low in fat, particularly saturated fat, which we know today is important in lowering the risk of heart disease. Certain of the current fad diets—e.g., the Atkins diet—are extremely high in fat and for this reason are potentially dangerous. The I Love New York Diet has adequate amounts of protein, but not too much like the Scarsdale or Stillman diets, and is high in fiber and other complex carbohydrates which we know today can protect against certain gastrointestinal problems. Finally, it is relatively low in salt, which may protect many susceptible people from high blood pressure.

But what is perhaps most important is that the Bureau of Nutrition realized that in order to really promote weight control, in order to help people lose weight and *keep it off*, patterns of eating had to be changed. The diet they developed was structured in such a way as to change people's eating habits for the rest of their lives. This remarkable branch of the New York City Health Department, a service that many New Yorkers don't even know exists, was twenty-five years ahead of the federal government. Only in 1979 did the U.S. Departments of Health and Human Services and of Agriculture publish guidelines for good nutrition. They are almost identical with this dietary scheme developed in New York City two and a half decades ago.

Unfortunately, as with many sensible and healthful ideas, the diet never received the publicity that it should have. While such nutritionally unsound eating plans as the Stillman, Atkins, Scarsdale, and Beverly Hills diets zoomed to the top of the best-seller lists by attracting thousands of people who had failed to lose weight on the diet they had tried before, the diet presented here was used only by those who contacted the Bureau of Nutrition or by those who heard about it by word of mouth.

The authors are providing a real service by publicizing this diet. Perhaps by naming the diet the I Love New York Diet they will give it enough style to make it widely used. I hope so. Perhaps the Bureau of Nutrition will get some of the recognition it so richly deserves. I hope so. Perhaps New York will become famous yet again for another first. I hope so. You see, I love New York.

MYRON WINICK, M.D.
Director, Institute of
Human Nutrition,
Columbia University, New York City

Contents

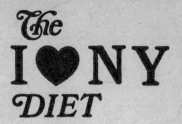

The
I ♥ NY
DIET

1

We've Got a Secret—
And We're Not Keeping
It to Ourselves

IF YOU ARE born and grow up in New York
City, you know right from the start about the exciting
variety of foods here.

If you come here to live or visit, you learn quickly
that one of the wonders of our wonderful town is that it
is an open invitation to an endlessly varied banquet.

No food is a stranger here. The countless restaurants
reflect every life-style and cultural background, which
combine to give New York its special touch among the
cities of the world.

Whether it's one of our many world-class restaurants,
or the little four-table place around the corner in the
neighborhood, or all the infinite decors and menus in
between, you are always within a short walk to those
foods which could only have been born in New York, or
to regional dishes from every part of our own country,

or to any of the more popular or almost unknown cuisines of the world.

But the restaurants are only part of it. The food shops reflect our sense of adventure in eating, and there's rarely a new product that doesn't attract shopper interest.

Along with that, we are a population that eats on the run. A fast pace breeds fast-food establishments. In addition, you can hardly walk down any street without encountering dozens of food carts on every block, offering every traditional or exotic food delight known to the palate of humankind.

The temptations are great. And for those who approach the banquet without discipline and common sense about nutrition, the penalties may also be great— a pain in the neck or any other part of the anatomy where excess pounds accumulate, or in the way in which too many of the wrong foods can conspire to be a costly and disquieting health menace to the unwary eater.

A sensible diet is the obvious and logical answer. Obvious and logical, but not easy. Too many obstacles are placed in the way between the potential dieter and the sensible diet.

Most dangerous of all the obstacles is the proliferation today of all the fad diets, many of which fly in the face of sensible nutrition, offering "magic" solutions to people desperate for better answers—and perhaps, in their vulnerability, too eager for the promised results to look closely at whether the exaggerated claims are substantiated. Betting on an unproven fad diet is like betting on a three-card monte game run by a street hustler—with your health and well-being as the ante.

Bill Adler and I don't like those odds. That's why we've joined together to bring you this book about a diet that has no "magic," but does have the nutritional sense that can work for you if you have the discipline to make it work.

It works already for many New Yorkers—and if it works here in this city of overwhelming eating temptations, it will work everywhere, for everyone.

Bill and I came to the diet by separate roads. I learned of it while I was Commissioner of Consumer Affairs of New York City and we were trying to do something about wider distribution of basic nutritional information. It didn't happen as successfully as we wanted it to happen, because our small Department, and the even smaller city Department that developed the diet, had neither the funds nor the capacity for a publicity blitz such as the fad diets mount today.

But the diet and I became inseparable. It's helped me to keep in shape and to maintain a high level of energy. The most recent time it came to my rescue was during my campaign for the United States Senate. Any campaign is a disrupter of regular hours and regular meals, and by the end of it I was a candidate for nutritional rehabilitation, and again the good sense of the diet helped me get rid of the bad habits of my recent experience.

That was the awareness of the diet that I brought with me when Bill Adler and I met during the course of some event around town. I hadn't seen Bill for a while, and I hadn't seen this particular Bill Adler for an even longer while. There was less of him, pounds less. All those pounds that a hard-working agent, spending endless hours sitting at his desk, slaving over a hot manuscript, with an abundance of snacks within reach, and exercising nothing except his editorial privilege, can accumulate until his office chair gradually becomes a much tighter fit.

"You look great, Bill," I said.

And then listened for a half hour to an enthusiastic tale of how Bill had discovered the diet which produced such pleasing results, which I quickly recognized as my own diet. In the face of such enthusiasm, all I could do was nod my head in agreement and mumble, "I know, I know."

"I had tried them all," Bill was saying, "the high-fat, the low-fat, the grapefruit, the everything-but-grapefruit, the calories-don't-count, the calories-do-count, the martini, the eat-everything, the eat-nothing. If it calls itself a diet, I've tried it. None of them worked."

"I know, I know," I said.

"I had heard about the diet of the New York City Department of Health," Bill continued, "and finally I called up the Bureau of Nutrition there, and asked what they recommended."

That's when he learned of the diet that the Bureau had worked out, a safe and sane diet that was successful and highly recommended by more doctors and research scientists than any diet in existence.

"The information has been available," Bill said, "but I

think more people should know about it. Everybody should know about it."

We looked at each other then, intensely. If we had been characters in a cartoon, that would have been the moment when the electric light over our heads lit up.

That's how the I Love New York Diet book began.

Before we began to assemble it, we conducted an informal survey to find out how much of a secret the diet really was, and what had been the experiences of some who had tried it.

We found out that many New Yorkers had discovered it and benefited from it. Some had been guided to it by their personal physicians, some had learned of it by word of mouth from their friends, some like Bill had had the initiative and good sense to go directly to the Bureau of Nutrition and ask for help. But some New Yorkers still haven't heard of the diet.

The comments we received from those for whom it was not a secret matched the enthusiasm Bill and I shared.

A network TV anchorwoman: "I was in danger of losing my job because I was fighting the battle of the bulge, and losing. With this diet I lost twelve and a half pounds in a very brief time. It works—and I'm working!"

A Park Avenue psychologist: "I went from 250 pounds to 170 pounds in just seven weeks. Waist size, 42 to 34. Suit size, 48 to 42. Collar size, 18½ to 16. Sorry, your hour is up."

A best-selling author, unhappy with the 158 pounds on her five foot four frame: "It was easy. It made sense.

And it was safe. I went down to 120 pounds in just three weeks. I followed the directions, and the diet did the rest."

A leading dancer: "I was in trouble. Extra weight and professional dancing don't go well together. I knew I had to get those pounds off. But I was afraid at first because I'd been through some of those other diets, and every one of them made me tired and irritable, and that shows in a performance. This one worked. The weight came off. And I felt great. Gave a great performance, too. I love that diet."

"It works." "It was safe." "It made sense." "And I felt great." Those words were part of the comments of everyone with whom we spoke, and the response buttressed our determination to make sure the word got out to greater numbers of people.

If we needed any more convincing, it came from the medical reports on the diet.

When Dr. Norman Jolliffe, former director of the Bureau of Nutrition, New York City Department of Health, researched and developed the diet, he issued an open invitation to New Yorkers to volunteer to help them test the new diet under the most rigorous scientific conditions before it would be announced to the general public.

More than 1,100 volunteers with various dietary and nutritional problems responded. The tests were conducted by a distinguished research team which, in addition to Dr. Jolliffe, included Dr. Seymour Rinzler and Morton Archer, a medical statistician. Of the more than 1,100 volunteers, most lost the desired amount of weight within a comparatively short period, and a larger percent than usual maintained their desired weight. Their general health improved, their energy was at a higher level, and—as one of the doctors expressed it—all in all, they were a more amiable group when the testing ended than they were before it began.

In another test not connected with the Bureau, Dr. Ancel Keys, one of our country's leading nutritionists, checked the diet on his own overweight patients. His conclusion: "It's perfectly safe, is not expensive, and can be taken with no sacrifice in longtime eating pleasure. I believe it's wise to accept it."

Dr. Leon Small, of the School of Medicine, George Washington University, conducted his own testing of the diet on a significant number of families. His report stated: "This dietary regime was readily acceptable by the family and required no change in the family diet habits."

Dr. Arthur Blumenfeld, a pioneer in diet nutrition, said after extensive testing: "This diet will not only add years to our lives, but more important, it can add vitality to our years." Dr. Seymour Rinzler added that it was an "easy" diet to follow and stay with.

That's the background which makes it so pleasing to me to be part of this book.

My own experiences with the diet, the dedication and impeccable honesty of the nutritionists in the New York City Department of Health, the support of responsible and respected medical authorities, the proven results for many New Yorkers—ranging from jet-setters in the headlines to anonymous hard-working men and women—and last, but certainly never least, the opportunity to work on the book with Bill Adler.

Bill is a concerned man and a highly respected member of the publishing profession, with a deep sense of responsibility both personally and professionally.

You have never seen his name on a fad diet book, and you never will. Because he did not believe in *The Beverly Hills Diet*, he turned it down. That's an old-fashioned virtue called principle.

That's the spirit and hope behind this book. That life-enhancing diet truths will reach as many people as possible, to clear away any confusions created by the fad diets and any nutritional con men who have found their way into the marketplace. To gather together in one handy book of plain language a diet that up to now has been scattered in mimeographed releases, hard-to-find scientific papers, and very sotto voce word of mouth.

In the pages that follow you'll learn about *our* diet—Bill's and mine—which is based on the nutritional principles of the Bureau of Nutrition's diet, and on the forerunners of that diet—Dr. Norman Jolliffe's Prudent Diet and his Reduce and Stay Reduced Diet. Our diet is fast, it's fun, and it works.

We call it the I Love New York Diet because it represents our city at its concerned best; but it's a diet for anyone, anywhere. No special foods are required, and no special preparations are needed. You can stay on this diet equally well in a restaurant or in your own home. And what you'll be eating is so similar to most of what you've been eating all along that you may have to wear a string around your finger to remind yourself you're really on a diet.

Bill and I can keep a secret as well as anyone—but not this one.

Don't wait until tomorrow to start your new diet. Turn over a new leaf, and start right now.

2

Why the I Love New York Diet Is the Only Diet You'll Ever Need

THE PERFECT DIET will slim you down to desired weight with the speed you demand and take you off the weight yo-yo once and for all.

The goal of the scientists at the Bureau of Nutrition, New York City Department of Health, was to develop the perfect diet. Their work was carried on in the same spirit that built the first atom bomb and sent astronauts to the moon. The creation of a perfect diet, many nutritionists have told us, is a feat comparable to those other two breakthrough scientific achievements.

In blueprinting the *I Love New York Diet*, we took the human equation—your special needs—into consideration. You can succeed only on a diet that produces results at once, is simple to follow, makes all the decisions for you, lasts the shortest possible time, doesn't disrupt your eating patterns or your daily life, is pleasant to be on—and ends calorie counting forever. On such a diet you can overcome the urge to overeat, raid the fridge, and chain-snack—without exerting the least bit of self-discipline. The perfect diet is for people like you and me who hate to work at dieting.

THE I LOVE NEW YORK DIET DOES EVERYTHING YOU'VE ALWAYS WANTED A DIET TO DO BUT NO DIET EVER DID BEFORE

It does this with seven spectacularly successful features:

1. *Immediate and rapid weight loss.* If you've never dieted before, the first anxious question you'll ask yourself is *"Can* I do it?" If you've ever dieted before, you know the answer is "Yes, I can do it—but only if I'm encouraged by quick results."

A top advertising exec, who called herself "a perpetual diet dropout" until she lost 11¼ pounds during the first week of the I Love New York Diet, said, "On other diets when I could see no results on my scale in the first few days, I would throw up my hands and wail, 'Oh, what's the use!' and give up. But on this miracle of a diet, I lost two pounds the *first* day, then *another two pounds* the second day, then *another two pounds* the third day, and I was hooked."

A basketball superstar, who had two weeks to remove twenty pounds of blubber before reporting to training camp, said, "I never thought I'd be able to stick to any diet. But when I saw those pounds just melting away day after day after day, man, I felt like I was on a hot streak. And when you're hot, man, you'd just be plain nuts to stop." He came into camp in midseason shape.

2. *Utter simplicity.* It's the simplest diet ever created.

3. *Freedom from decision making.* This diet tells you what to eat, when to eat it, and even how to eat it. Nothing is left to chance. All you have to do is follow simple instructions to the letter.

As an overweight you can do that better than most other people, according to a study made by Dr. Ian MacBurney, a psychologist specializing in diet problems. "Fatties," he concluded, "are superior people. [But] brightness isn't the only trait that places you a notch or two above the general population. You're [also] a whiz at following instructions. When you're told to do something, you do it exactly right, and you do it right the first time."

On a diet the last thing you want to do is think about food. On this diet you don't have to. All the thinking has been done for you by experts.

4. *A one-week crash program.* No reducing program is shorter.

"When I'm told it will take me five weeks to lose ten pounds, forget it," a director of marketing at a leading department store confided. "Even a two-week or three-week program seems like it will never end. That's why I fell in love with the I Love New York Diet. I lost ten pounds in one week—and the week went by like lightning."

Dr. Norman Jolliffe, one of the creators of the I Love

New York Diet, reports weight losses in one week of up to ten pounds. Average one-week weight losses ranged from five to seven pounds. (Much of the weight lost during the first few days is fluid. Thereafter, fat begins to disappear.)

As a reward for losing so much weight so fast—a feat you can be proud of—you're treated to a one-week I Love New York Eating Holiday. You'll eat to your heart's content without gaining an ounce. You can even lose weight should you desire to do so.

If you're one of those people who find it difficult to remain with any diet for more than three or four days, the Eating Holiday is a powerful lure to keep you going. "Every time I found myself weakening after the third day," a discotheque owner told us as we admired her stunning new figure, "I said to myself, 'Only three more days to the Eating Holiday,' then, 'Only two more days,' then, 'Only one more day,' and—hurray!—for the first time in my life I made it!"

If at the end of your Eating Holiday you feel you should lose more weight—and many heavy people do— then go back to another exciting crash weight-loss week, and once again reward your remarkable success with a week's Eating Holiday. Alternate the Crash Program with the Eating Holiday as often as you like until you're down to your desired weight. It's easy to lose fifty, sixty, seventy pounds or more when you crash-diet for no more than one week at a time.

5. *Available in restaurants.* Anybody can lose weight under rigidly controlled clinical conditions, as on a fat farm or at a health spa. But this diet was constructed for quick, easy, and permanent weight loss in the real

world. You can go into most restaurants and order I Love New York Diet breakfasts, lunches, dinners, and even snacks. Forget about brown paper bags and carrying plastic packs of raw vegetables around with you all day. This is a practical diet which does not require you to alter your life-style in any way.

6. *You don't count calories.* "I hate calorie-counting diets," one of our jet-set friends declared. "When you have to eat with one eye on the menu and the other eye on your calorie counter, there's no joy left in dining. Eating is too pleasant a part of life to make it a bore or a chore."

That's why calorie counting is eliminated on the I Love New York Diet. Calories do count, of course, but all the calorie counting has been done for you. All you do is follow the simple instructions, and enjoy your food.

7. *Freedom from suffering.* One reason dieting has been dreaded up to now is that it can become one of the most painful experiences of anybody's life. Popular fad diets produce draggy and dizzy feelings; ketosis, a condition associated with diabetes, which is likely to cause weakness, nausea, vomiting, and foul breath; leg cramps; flagging energy; dry and scaly skin; diarrhea; and a host of other disagreeable side effects. Plus plain ordinary hunger and its accompanying psychological distress symptoms.

"I don't believe any dieting is painless," wrote diet expert Corinne T. Metzer.

Dr. H. L. Newbold, a nutrition expert, warned the would-be dieter, "You may feel miserable on the first seven or eight days of [any] diet."

But these comments were made without knowledge of the I Love New York Diet. Before we knew about this perfect diet, we would have agreed with them. Bill had gone through the agonies of dieting many times. But on this diet at no time did he become the cranky, irritable Mr. Hyde his wife and kids feared from his previous failures at shedding weight. There were no circles under his eyes, no hollows in his cheeks, no feelings of depression and fatigue. Best of all, there was no great void in his stomach or feelings of deprivation. He felt satisfied, energetic, and high-spirited. He was more vigorous than he had been when he wasn't dieting.

At long last, we had found a diet it was a pleasure to stay on. You'll find it a pleasure, too.

3

Three Nutritional Breakthroughs That Let You Shed Pounds, Look Shapelier, on a Full Stomach

As WE TRAVEL around the country, we find a rising tide of interest in healthful dieting, particularly among young people. They inform me that they want to undo the effect junk foods have had on them, and lead the rest of their lives with slim, vigorous bodies. Older people, too, are excited about the prospect of living healthier, longer, more active lives at their ideal weights. The interest of everybody not only covers the "how" of dieting, but also the "why."

"*Why* does it work? Is there some sort of magic ingredient?" people ask.

The only magic is the magic of scientific achievements. Not just one great scientific breakthrough but three were put to work by researchers who were responsible for the ultra-successful diets on which this diet is based. Here in plain language is what those

17

breakthroughs are all about; and "why," when combined into a single unique eating pattern, they cut your weight and improve your figure on a full stomach. (*Advice:* If you would rather get started on the diet than find out how it works, skip to the next chapter. Then while you watch your fat melting away, come back and get acquainted with the three great weight-loss breakthroughs that do it for you.)

THE FIRST GREAT WEIGHT-LOSS BREAKTHROUGH: *YOU CAN EAT YOUR FILL OF THE FOOD YOU LOVE*

Let's say, to get that filled-up feeling you need four portions of food, as illustrated by the following boxes:

C	P	F	F	
1	1	2	2	= 6

The numerals add up to 6. Let's also say that number 6 is keeping you fat; and should the numerals in the four portions add up to any number less than 6, you'll lose weight.

Losing weight then becomes very simple; You just substitute a 1-portion for a 2-portion.

C	P	P	F	
1	1	1	2	= 5

The numerals add up to 5. You're losing weight. But you still have the four portions that give you that filled-up feeling. You're actually losing weight on a full stomach!

The letter C stands for carbohydrate, a 1-portion; P for protein, a 1-portion; and F for fat, a 2-portion. The point is: *When you substitute a portion of protein (or carbohydrate) for a portion of fat, you lose weight, while the amount of food you consume remains the same.*

For the scientifically minded, the explanation is just as simple. One gram of fat contributes about two times the amount of calories as one gram of carbohydrate or protein. When you substitute a gram of carbohydrate or protein for a gram of fat, you ingest the same amount of food but you cut your caloric intake by 50 percent. When you cut calories, you drop weight.

The I Love New York Diet is a low-fat diet.

When the amount of fat you eat is reduced, your body, in order to operate efficiently, burns up your stored fat—all that ugly blubber you hate. Your excess fat simply disappears.

Good riddance! Any doctor will tell you that more fat than you need can lead to diabetes, high blood pressure, heart attack, and numerous other degenerative diseases. Any member of the opposite sex will tell you that excess fat means "No, no, a thousand times no!" And any personnel director will tell you that the response to superfluous fat is usually "Don't call us. We'll call you."

When you cut out fat in your diet, your appearance improves so much, people will think you've had a face- and body-lift. Aging, unsightly fat vanishes from under your chin and around your breasts, from your thighs, your upper arms, your shoulders, your buttocks, and your belly. A low-fat diet means a healthier, a sexier, and a more employable you.

But it does not mean a starving or a deprived you. You can eat your fill of steak, shrimp, turkey, roast beef, chicken, clams, fish, salads, fruit, and approved vegetables. You can drink all the tea and coffee you wish, all the low-calorie sodas, all the mineral water and tap water. You will feel well-nourished and satisfied every minute of the day. A low-fat diet is *the* diet every food lover has always dreamed about.

THE SECOND GREAT WEIGHT-LOSS BREAKTHROUGH: *YOU CAN LOSE INCHES, LOOK FITTER—FASTER*

That lovely lean look of your favorite fighter or ballerina comes from more muscle tissue and less fat tissue. You can get that look faster with this diet plus exercise than by exercise alone. Here's how the diet helps:

Dr. Norman Jolliffe, one of the researchers on whose work the I Love New York Diet is based, discovered that substituting high-value protein foods for fatty foods increases the amount of muscle tissue in your body while decreasing the amount of fat tissue. The diet provides your body with a head start when you exercise to trim off inches and look fitter. *That's why the I Love New York Diet is a low-fat diet which supplies generous amounts of protein.*

The I Love New York Diet and Exercise Program (page 173) not only slims you down, it helps shape you up.

THE THIRD GREAT WEIGHT-LOSS BREAKTHROUGH: *FIBER FILLS YOU UP*

The I Love New York Diet is above all practical. It takes all your eating needs into account. To most dieters the most urgent of those needs is the desire to snack.

On the I Love New York Diet, you can snack to your heart's content on foods that contain few or no calories but plenty of bulk. These are high-fiber foods.

Dr. Judith S. Stern of the Department of Nutrition, University of California, calls fiber a "miracle nutrient." She explains that fiber swells in the stomach, giving a feeling of satiety "so you won't be driven to eat more than you need to feel full." For that reason high-fiber foods—which include oranges, apples, asparagus, broccoli, and cauliflower—are also a major part of all I Love New York Diet meals.

That, finally, is the carefully calculated combination of nutrients that explains "why" this exceptional diet worked for those 1,100 human guinea pigs, and why it can work to transform you into the attractive new you you've always dreamed of becoming.

Fashionable New Yorkers agree that this nutritious mix does another wonderful thing. It gives you a sense of well-being, vigor, and a peace of mind that you never experienced before.

4

The Complete I Love New York Diet—The Easiest Diet Ever

NEW WE'RE GETTING down to the reality of dieting. "At this point," one three-time diet loser confessed, "I always shiver. I've always found dieting such hard, hard work."

Not any longer. This is a serious diet, not a fad diet, but it's a fun diet. It's like playing a game. Just follow these easy steps, and you'll agree with the prizewinning author who told us, "I didn't believe a diet could be so easy until I tried it myself."

THE I LOVE NEW YORK DIET BASIC RAPID-WEIGHT-LOSS PLAN

Step 1. Establish your weight goal. How many pounds do

CHART OF IDEAL WEIGHTS*

Height (feet and inches)	MEN light	Build medium	heavy	WOMEN light	Build medium	heavy
4-10	95	100	105	90	94	98
4-11	97	103	108	93	98	102
5-0	100	106	111	95	100	105
5-1	105	111	117	97	102	108
5-2	110	117	123	100	106	111
5-3	115	122	128	105	112	118
5-4	120	127	133	110	116	123
5-5	125	132	138	112	119	126
5-6	130	137	143	117	124	130
5-7	133	141	148	120	127	134
5-8	137	145	153	125	132	139
5-9	143	151	159	130	137	144
5-10	148	156	164	135	142	149
5-11	152	160	168	140	147	154
6-0	155	163	171	144	151	158
6-1	163	171	179			
6-2	167	175	183			
6-3	170	179	188			
6-4	172	181	195			
6-5	178	188	198			
6-6	185	195	206			

Reprinted with permission from *Diet for Life* by Francine Prince (New York, N.Y.: Cornerstone Library, Inc., 1981).

*This table applies to men and women age twenty-five or older. If you're eighteen to twenty-five, subtract one pound for every year you're under twenty-five.

you want to lose? That's up to you. "I know I'm still a bit—well—pleasantly plump," the chef at a posh Manhattan restaurant, who had lost thirty-nine pounds on the I Love New York Diet, said. "But I feel comfortable this way. I don't think my customers would have confidence in me if I looked thin and scrawny." Whatever weight makes you comfortable is the right weight for you.

Many people say to us, "I would just like to be average weight." They're under the illusion that average weight is the best weight. It's not. The average weight represents the weight of all the adults in the United States divided by their total number. Since most adults are overweight, when you're at average weight you're overweight.

The best weight is the ideal weight. That's the one at which Americans are healthiest and live longest, according to insurance-company statistics. The ideal weight is about ten to fifteen pounds less than the average weight.

Have you decided on your weight-loss goal? Good! Now go on to Step 2.

Step 2. Cut out the 7-Day Crash Program Scoreboard, which appears on the following page, and tape it on your full-length mirror at eye level.

Step 3. Begin the I Love New York Diet on any day of the week. (Details of the diet begin on page 33).

On the day you choose, weigh yourself naked before breakfast. (If you don't have a bathroom scale, run out

THE I LOVE NEW YORK DIET
7-DAY CRASH PROGRAM
SCOREBOARD

YOUR WEIGHT

☐

Present Weight

DAYS ON DIET		DAILY WEIGHT LOSS
1	☐	☐
2	☐	☐
3	☐	☐
4	☐	☐
5	☐	☐
6	☐	☐
7	☐	☐

NEW SLIMMED-DOWN WEIGHT _____

☐

**WEIGHT LOSS
IN JUST ONE
WEEK**

and get one.) Enter your weight in the box above "Present Weight."

On the morning of the second day, weigh yourself *at the same time as you did the day before*. You've now been on the diet for one day, so enter your weight in the appropriate box on the same line as the numeral 1. Here's an example:

YOUR WEIGHT

161

Present Weight

DAYS ON DIET **DAILY WEIGHT LOSS**

1 159

Now subtract your new weight from your weight the day before and enter the result in the empty box under "Daily Weight Loss."

YOUR WEIGHT

161

Present Weight

DAYS ON DIET **DAILY WEIGHT LOSS**

1 159 2

I (Bill) had lost two pounds the very first day! What a grand and glorious feeling! I felt as good as when I make a major book sale for one of my clients. I couldn't wait to read the scale the next day. As soon as I did, I rushed to the scoreboard with a song in my heart and entered the numbers.

YOUR WEIGHT

161

Present Weight

DAYS ON DIET		DAILY WEIGHT LOSS
1	159	2
2	157	2

I had lost four pounds in just two days! I stepped back and looked at myself in the full-length mirror on which I had taped my *7-Day Crash Program Scoreboard*. I was perceptibly trimmer! And I felt much lighter. Four pounds doesn't seem like much, but it's a lot of weight when you have to carry it around all day long. Fill a plastic bag with four pounds of fat and lug it with you for a full day without putting it down once, and you'll understand what I mean. I felt good, encouraged. I looked forward eagerly to the next day's reading.

I lost only one pound. No, it was not a disappointment. I knew from reading case histories of people on the I Love New York Diet that losing weight is not governed by a mathematical equation but by the human equation. I knew that because of such variables as stress, energy expenditure, and emotional activities, my daily weight losses could fluctuate. Some days I could lose one pound, some days one and a half pounds, some days two pounds, and some days more. Losing just one pound was no setback. Besides, I had lost five pounds in only three days, and that was marvelous. Feeling happy and excited, I continued on the diet. My scoreboard, as it looked after one week, appears on the following page.

It's a winner's scoreboard. It represents the easiest victory I ever had achieved in my life. All I did was follow simple instructions. On the I Love New York Diet anybody can become a winner the same way. The lighter, shapelier person you meet in your mirror after the first week will agree.

Here's a plus: If you only have to knock off a few pounds, you can do it in just a few days.

Step 4. Reward yourself for your spectacular weight-loss achievement with a one-week I Love New York Eating Holiday. The mouth-watering details begin on page 51. At the end of your Eating Holiday week, you'll be as thin as, or thinner than, you were at the end of your first diet week.

Should you then desire to lose more weight, return to the crash I Love New York Diet for as many weeks as you need. But never stay on the diet for more than one

YOUR WEIGHT

161

Present Weight

DAYS ON DIET		DAILY WEIGHT LOSS
1	159	2
2	157	2
3	156	1
4	155	1
5	152	3
6	151	1
7	150	1

NEW SLIMMED-DOWN WEIGHT _____ 150

11

**WEIGHT LOSS
IN JUST ONE
WEEK**

week at a time. After each week, reward yourself with a one-week Eating Holiday.

While you're dieting and while you're on your Eating Holiday, make entries on the appropriate scoreboard every day. You'll find an ample supply of scoreboards beginning on page 209.

Step 5. After you've slimmed down to your desired weight, stay thin effortlessly on the I Love New York Lifetime Stay-Slim Program. In tests conducted by the Bureau of Nutrition, New York City Department of Health, this healthfully delicious way of eating all the food you want while maintaining your desired weight was successful in almost every case.

That's all there is to it!

Start tomorrow on the easiest diet *ever.* And take those excess pounds off *forever.*

5

The 7-Day Crash Program: Drop Ten Pounds or More —Automatically

HERE ARE SEVEN DAYS of complete rapid-weight-loss menus. They take into account the current practice of eating seven times a day—three major meals, two coffee breaks, a TV snack, and a bedtime snack.

Important:

These menus will take off your excess weight rapidly and automatically. That's because powerful fat-destroying principles are built into the diet. But they will not work unless you follow the menus and the related instructions *exactly as written*. Do not deviate in any way. Do not add, subtract, or substitute a single item. And never under any circumstance skip a meal.

Here are your basic instructions. They're designed to make dieting a pleasure.

THE THREE I LOVE NEW YORK DIET RULES FOR EATING ENJOYMENT

1. Eat slowly to savor every morsel.
2. Eat everything (except for a few quantity-limited foods) until you're satisfied.
3. Don't stuff yourself; it will make you feel uncomfortable.

Now enjoy your first I Love New York Diet breakfast. Thousands of fashionable New Yorkers are enjoying it, too.

THE I LOVE NEW YORK ONE-WEEK CRASH DIET MENUS

FIRST DAY

BREAKFAST
Orange
Egg, boiled or poached
Piece Melba toast
Coffee or tea

MORNING COFFEE BREAK
Approved snacks and beverages (page 42)

LUNCH
Shrimp or seafood of your choice
Celery, lettuce, tomato, and carrot sticks
Coffee, tea, or diet soda

AFTERNOON COFFEE BREAK
Approved snacks and beverages

DINNER
Fresh fruit cocktail
Sautéed chicken breasts
Cabbage, turnips, and zucchini (or Brussels sprouts)
Coffee, tea, or club soda with lemon or lime

TV SNACK
Approved beverages and snacks

BEDTIME SNACK
Cup low-fat milk

SECOND DAY

BREAKFAST
   Grapefruit
   Cottage cheese (or low-fat pot cheese)
   Coffee or tea

MORNING COFFEE BREAK
   Approved snacks and beverages

LUNCH
   Sliced roast beef
   Lettuce, celery, and tomato
   Coffee, tea, or diet soda

AFTERNOON COFFEE BREAK
   Approved snacks and beverages

DINNER
   Tomato juice or V-8 (preferably with no salt added)
   Broiled liver
   Spinach, cauliflower, celery, and green pepper
   Coffee, tea, or club soda with lemon or lime

TV SNACK
   Approved beverages and snacks

BEDTIME SNACK
   Cup low-fat milk

THIRD DAY

BREAKFAST
Orange
Puffed wheat (preferably with no salt added)
Low-fat milk
Coffee or tea

MORNING COFFEE BREAK
Approved snacks and beverages

LUNCH
Fresh fruit salad
Cottage cheese
Coffee, tea, or diet soda

AFTERNOON SNACK
Approved snacks and beverages

DINNER
Clams
Flounder, haddock, or fish of your choice
Celery, radishes, carrots, and zucchini (or cabbage)
Coffee, tea, or club soda with lemon or lime

TV SNACK
Approved snacks and beverages

BEDTIME SNACK
Cup low-fat milk

FOURTH DAY

BREAKFAST
Grapefruit
Shredded wheat
Low-fat milk
Coffee or tea

MORNING COFFEE BREAK
Approved snacks and beverages

LUNCH
Canned fish, such as tuna (oil removed, or packed in
water or broth)
Lettuce, cucumbers, celery, and radishes
Coffee, tea, or club soda with lemon or lime

AFTERNOON COFFEE BREAK
Approved snacks and beverages

DINNER
Roast veal
Mixed green salad
Strawberries or other berries in season
Coffee, tea, or club soda with lemon or lime

TV SNACK
Approved snacks and beverages

BEDTIME SNACK
Cup low-fat milk

FIFTH DAY

BREAKFAST
Tangerine or orange
½ thin slice bread
Low-fat milk
Coffee or tea

MORNING SNACK
Approved snacks and beverages

LUNCH
Broiled hamburger
Green salad with sliced tomatoes
Coffee, tea, or diet soda

AFTERNON SNACK
Approved snacks and beverages

DINNER
Broiled chicken
Asparagus, spinach, and cauliflower
Fresh fruit salad
Coffee, tea, or club soda with lemon or lime

TV SNACK
Approved snacks and beverages

BEDTIME SNACK
Cup low-fat milk

SIXTH DAY

BREAKFAST
  Grapefruit
  Egg, boiled or poached
  Piece RyKrisp
  Coffee or tea

MORNING COFFEE BREAK
  Approved snacks and beverages

LUNCH
  Chicken or turkey slices
  Lettuce, celery, and tomatoes
  Coffee, tea, or diet soda

AFTERNOON COFFEE BREAK
  Approved snacks and beverages

DINNER
  Steak or London broil
  Broccoli, string beans, and green peppers
  Strawberries
  Coffee, tea, or club soda with lemon or lime

TV SNACK
  Approved snacks and beverages

BEDTIME SNACK
  Cup low-fat milk

SEVENTH DAY

BREAKFAST
  Orange
  Shredded wheat
  Low-fat milk
  Coffee or tea

MORNING COFFEE BREAK
  Approved snacks and beverages

LUNCH
  Sliced hard-cooked eggs
  Mixed green salad
  Coffee, tea, or diet soda

AFTERNOON COFFEE BREAK
  Approved snacks and beverages

DINNER
  Crabmeat or seafood of your choice
  Spinach, broccoli, and carrots
  Grapefruit
  Coffee, tea, or club soda with lemon or lime

TV SNACK
  Approved snacks and beverages

BEDTIME SNACK
  Cup low-fat milk

APPROVED SNACKS

- All the raw vegetables you can eat, especially broccoli, carrots, green and red peppers, celery, cauliflower, radishes, cucumbers, and turnip slices.
- 1 tablespoon sesame seeds.
- All the coffee, tea, diet soda, club soda, mineral water, or tap water you can drink.

6

How to Make the I Love New York Diet Work for You at Top Speed

You can go through the seven days of rapid-weight-loss menus, then gaze at yourself in a full-length mirror and at the numbers on your scoreboard with rapturous amazement. But if you know a few "tricks of the trade"—up-to-the-minute nutritional and psychological aids to dieting—which few dieters are aware of, you can drop an additional three pounds a week or more. You can even overcome your natural "mañana" attitude and get started on the diet at once.

Here is a roundup of aids for faster dieting presented as answers to questions most frequently asked.

I need to diet and I want to diet, but I keep putting it off and putting it off and putting it off. What shall I do?

Motivate yourself psychologically in one or more of the following ways:

1. Tell everybody you know that you're going on a diet—and the exact day you're going on it. Then if you don't go on it and stay on it, and you'll get those I-knew-you-couldn't-do-it looks. It's less painful to *do* it, particularly on the painless I Love New York Diet.

2. Tell yourself you're going to enjoy the most memorable week in your life—the week in which you become, or start to become, the person you always wanted to be. Picture yourself slipping into a size 8 for the first time in twenty years; or if you're a man, wearing a thirty-inch belt again. All the others in your set will eat their hearts out. That's worth getting started at once, isn't it?

3. Look at your first diet week as an adventure, a challenge, an exciting relief from your daily humdrum activities. While your spouse, friends and relatives, and the people you work with watch in amazement as the pounds melt away, you'll become a star. Why delay?

4. Remind yourself that you have only one short week to go before you can revel in an Eating Holiday. If you're fortyish, you've already gone through about 2,000 weeks. What's just one week more, particularly when each day brings you closer to one of the great eating experiences of your lifetime? The sooner you get started, the sooner you'll get to it.

And—

5. Repeat to yourself over and over again: Fat is unattractive, unhealthy, aging, unfashionable. The only way to get that unpleasant refrain out of your head is to go on the I Love New York Diet, and stay on it.

Will exercise speed up weight loss?

Certainly. If you're under forty-five and your doctor gives you a clean bill of health, strenuous exercise is okay if you enjoy it. If you don't, why don't you do what Bill does? He walks briskly to and from his office—more than four miles a day, six days a week. If you're not used to walking, start with a half a mile a day, then increase it gradually to one mile, then to two miles. Walk briskly two miles a day, and you'll shed an extra half pound a week.

Exercise has another advantage. It replaces fatty tissue, which is bulky and blubbery, with muscle tissue, which is compact and streamlined. Exercise helps you get that firm, fit look of the celebrities in *People* magazine.

But as Dr. Lloyd C. Arnold, National Director of Health and Physical Education, National Board of the YMCA, warns, conditioning yourself just on weekends "doesn't work very well. No [end-of-the-week] surge of effort can replace a daily lifestyle that includes some ...exercise."

I'm a European and I'm accustomed to eating my salad before my meat, fish, or poultry. But on the menus, salads are listed after those dishes. Must I eat them in that order?

Actually, eating salad *before* your main course is better than eating it *with* the main course or *after* it. Salad is a hunger killer, provided the dressing is not packed with salt, an appetite stimulator. We recommend that vegetables as well as salad greens be eaten before your main

45

course. These low, low-calorie foods will take the edge off your desire for higher-calorie meat, poultry, and fish. You'll save hundreds of calories a day, which can mean an extra pound or so lost by the end of the week.

What kind of dressing should I use on my salad?

None is best. You'll experience, perhaps for the first time in your life, the natural goodness of fresh greens. But if you insist on a dressing, oil and vinegar are preferable with the accent on vinegar. Or make your own dressing—it's easy—by mixing corn oil and your choice of herb vinegar. For gourmets recipes have been included for virtually no-cal salad dressings, based on those devised by Dr. Norman Jolliffe. You'll find them on pages 132, 147, and 148. Recommended salad dressings speed up your weight loss; commercial dressings slow it down.

May I put sugar and whole milk or cream in my coffee?

Not if you want to reduce fast. But to any kind of coffee—from instant to espresso—you can add a non-caloric sweetener and low-fat milk. The flavor of coffee is also perked up by cinnamon (use it in stick form) and lemon rind. Sugar is highly caloric; and so is whole milk, which is extremely fatty to boot. The same guidelines apply to tea.

We prepare fish and vegetables at home with plenty of butter and salt. Is that the right way to do it?

Sorry, it's the wrong way. Butter is a high-calorie fat; and salt helps retain excess body water, which shows up on your scale. By eliminating butter in cooking and as a spread, and by holding the salt you use—in cooking and from the salt shaker—to a minimum, you can easily drop an extra two or three pounds a week. Use herbs and spices instead. They're calorie-free.

May I use margarine instead of butter?

Not on the reducing diet. Margarine is 100 percent fat, and has as many calories as butter. Diet margarine is okay on the maintenance diet, but it adds too many calories to the reducing diet.

Why aren't ketchup, pickles, and relishes on the menus? They have very few calories.

True. But they do have a great deal of salt, which can increase blood pressure in some people. Salt also retains water and water means added weight.

The menus call for broiled fish and sautéed chicken breasts. I like fried foods. Any objection?

Yes, indeed. Fried foods retain a large amount of the frying fats. When you broil, excess fat drips away. Sautéing uses only a minimum of fat in a conventional skillet, and none at all in a non-stick skillet. Broiling and sautéing are the cooking techniques preferred for quick weight loss.

The menus call for meat, poultry, and fish. On my plate I can see the fat, sometimes even on fish. Am I supposed to eat it?

Never eat the fat. When eating in restaurants, trim away all visible fat and discard it. When eating at home, trim away all visible fat from meat and fish before cooking. Do the same with chicken and also remove the skin. The skin contains at least 25 percent of the fat content of a chicken. For faster weight reduction, never eat chicken skin.

May I substitute canned foods for the fresh foods on the menu?

Canned foods are usually packed with salt and sugar (read the labels), which are no-no's on a reducing diet. Salt adds unnecessary water weight, and sugar unneeded calories. The only acceptable canned food on the Crash Program is tuna. You can speed up weight reduction by using a "dietetic" pack or by draining the oil from the regular pack.

May I substitute frozen foods for fresh foods?

Frozen foods are acceptable when fresh foods are not available, except when added salt content is high. Salt is designated as "sodium in milligrams per serving." When the sodium content tops 200 milligrams, don't buy. Let the label be your guide.

On the menus no specific quantities are given for steak, fish, chicken, salads, vegetables, and snacks. Does that really mean I can eat all I want until I feel full?

Yes. But you'll lose weight faster when you follow these anti-overeating guidelines:

- When you're eating at home, serve yourself normal restaurant-sized portions. Do not serve family style.

- Leave one tenth of your food on the plate.

- Drink approved beverages just before and during your meals, not after.

- Drink plenty of water and approved beverages between meals.

I never eat breakfast. Won't I lose weight faster if I continue to skip it?

No way. You'll just be so much hungrier at coffee breaks and lunchtimes that you'll go off the diet.

I don't like some of the food on the menus. What substitutions can I make?

None. Food preferences are acquired tastes, and you can get to like anything. Bill was no cottage-cheese fan when he went on this diet, but now he eats it with gusto. The whole point of sticking to the diet exactly as written is *it will take weight off you fast.* Any deviation, no matter how small, will slow you down.

And here's a plus: You're building new taste preferences that will help keep you slim and attractive for the rest of your life.

But there are exceptions. If, because of health or religious reasons, you cannot eat some of the prescribed food, or if some of the prescribed food is not available, make commonsense substitutions. For example, pork can be replaced with veal or lamb (lean cuts, please).

7

Take an I Love New York Eating Holiday

You've come to the end of the first week on the I Love New York Diet. Your scoreboard shows a loss of ten pounds or more. You look fantastic in your full-length mirror. It's time to celebrate. Bring on the champagne!

Yes, *champagne*.

Or any other alcoholic beverage you like.

"Then why couldn't I have a drink the first week?" people often ask.

You're getting very few calories during that first week, even though your stomach doesn't know it. So to keep up your strength—in fact, to make you feel better and more vigorous than ever—every calorie of food has to be crammed with nutritive value. A calorie of alcohol has no nutritive value at all. That's why alcohol was banned from the Crash Diet we developed.

But liquor, especially wine, has been accepted medically since biblical times as a safe and powerful potion for lifting your spirits and giving you a sense of well-being when used in moderation. "A day without wine," goes an old French proverb, "is like a day without sunshine." On the I Love New York Eating Holiday, you can have a glass of wine (not sweet), a jigger of hard liquor, a bottle of beer, or a cocktail (without sugar) once a day. You don't have to have it, but if you want it—enjoy it. This week is a reward for your sensational achievement of last week, and liquor can be part of the fun.

GO ON A CONTROLLED BINGE WHILE KEEPING YOUR WEIGHT STEADY OR CONTINUING TO LOSE

On your Eating Holiday you'll be enjoying potatoes, pasta, blue-cheese dressing, bread and rolls, rice, beef stew, chopped liver, peanut butter, commercial breakfast cereals, margarine, your favorite cheeses, cole slaw, condiments, and cakes and desserts. Yet you won't gain an ounce, and you could lose several pounds.

This is a controlled binge. It satisfies every dieter's craving for familiar food, and lots of it, without on-the-scale regrets. "A wonderful thing about the Eating Holiday," a young actress said, "is that you *feel* you're on a binge, but you feel no guilt because the food is so slimming and so good for you. I wouldn't mind binging like this for the rest of my life."

Your basic instructions are the same as for the first week:

THE THREE I LOVE NEW YORK DIET RULES FOR EATING ENJOYMENT

1. Eat slowly to savor every morsel.
2. Eat everything (except for a few quantity-limited foods) until you're satisfied.
3. Don't stuff yourself; it will make you feel uncomfortable.

And to make your Eating Holiday work better for you, follow these guidelines:

· Remember to take it easy with the salt shaker, and go light on pickles and other salty condiments. You'll be able to eat more food when you eat less salt. (Salt clings to water, and water is heavy.)

· Make use of all the diet aids you learned about in the preceding chapter.

· Use liquid vegetable oils of your choice for salads and cooking.

53

THE I LOVE NEW YORK
EATING HOLIDAY
SCOREBOARD

YOUR WEIGHT

Present Weight

DAYS ON DIET		DAILY WEIGHT LOSS
1		
2		
3		
4		
5		
6		
7		

NEW SLIMMED-DOWN WEIGHT _____

**WEIGHT LOSS
IN JUST ONE
WEEK**

- Spread margarine in a thin layer on your bread or potatoes. You'll be amazed how much better it tastes that way. Diet margarine is preferred.

- Weigh yourself every day before breakfast, and enter your weight on *The I Love New York Eating Holiday Scoreboard* (there's one on the facing page), which you've taped up on your full-length mirror at eye level.

THE I LOVE NEW YORK EATING HOLIDAY MENUS

FIRST DAY

BREAKFAST
Pineapple juice
Slice whole-wheat toast with margarine (diet margarine preferred)
Cream of wheat
Low-fat milk
Raisins
Coffee or tea

MORNING COFFEE BREAK
Approved snacks and soft drinks.

LUNCH
Grapefruit juice
Canned mackerel

Mixed green salad with dressing of your choice
Bread
Pickles and condiments (optional)
Any approved soft drink

AFTERNOON COFFEE BREAK
Approved snacks and soft drinks

DINNER
Cocktail, had liquor, beer, or wine (optional)
Chicken with noodles
Green peas
Eggplant salad
Whole-grain bread
Pickles and condiments (optional)
Melon (if not in season, any other fresh fruit)
Coffee, tea, or club soda with lemon or lime

TV SNACK
Popcorn (unsalted)

BEDTIME SNACK
Cup low-fat milk

SECOND DAY

BREAKFAST
Orange
Canadian bacon
Slice toast with margarine
Coffee or tea

MORNING COFFEE BREAK
Approved snacks and soft drinks

LUNCH
Tomato juice
Chef's salad, composed of hard-cooked eggs, lean
    ham, chicken, and dressing of your choice
Pickles and condiments (optional)
Sponge cake
Any approved soft drink

AFTERNOON COFFEE BREAK
Approved snacks and soft drinks

DINNER
Cocktail, hard liquor, beer, or wine (optional)
Baked fish
Salad composed of pasta shells, cooked greens, and
    dressing of your choice
Fresh fruit cup
Coffee, tea, or club soda with lemon or lime

TV SNACK
Dates and cheese chunks

BEDTIME SNACK
Cup low-fat milk

THIRD DAY

BREAKFAST
Orange
Hot oatmeal
Low-fat milk
Coffee or tea

MORNING COFFEE BREAK
Approved snacks and soft drinks

LUNCH
Tomato juice
Lean sliced beef
Lettuce wedges with salad dressing of your choice
Slice rye bread with margarine
Pickles and condiments (optional)
Angel food cake
Any approved soft drink

AFTERNOON COFFEE BREAK
Approved snacks and soft drinks

DINNER
Cocktail, hard liquor, beer, or wine (optional)
Broiled fish
Potato salad
Cooked greens
Corn bread with margarine
Coffee, tea, or club soda with lemon or lime

TV SNACK
Raisins and walnuts

FOURTH DAY

BREAKFAST
Grapefruit juice
Wheat flakes
Low-fat milk
Swiss cheese
Slice toast
Coffee or tea

MORNING COFFEE BREAK
Approved snacks and beverages

LUNCH
Tomato juice
Chopped liver
2 slices rye bread
Cucumbers and radishes
Pickles and condiments (optional)
Baked apple
Any approved soft drink

AFTERNOON COFFEE BREAK
Approved snacks and soft drinks

DINNER
Cocktail, hard liquor, beer, or wine (optional)
Lean pork with bean sprouts

Brown rice
Spinach
Hard roll
Pickles and condiments (optional)
Pineapple cubes (fresh or packed in own juice)
Coffee, tea, or club soda with lemon or lime

TV SNACK
Figs and cheese chunks

BEDTIME SNACK
Cup low-fat milk

FIFTH DAY

BREAKFAST
Blend of orange and grapefruit juice
Any ready-to-eat breakfast cereal
Low-fat milk
Slice toast with margarine
Coffee or tea

MORNING COFFEE BREAK
Approved snacks and soft drinks

LUNCH
Tuna salad with dressing of your choice
Mixed raw vegetables
Slice whole-wheat bread with margarine
Pickles and condiments (optional)

Sherbet
Any approved soft drink

AFTERNOON COFFEE BREAK
Approved snacks and soft drinks

DINNER
Cocktail, hard liquor, beer, or wine (optional)
Red beans and rice
Tomato salad with dressing of your choice
Slice bread with margarine
Fresh fruit cup
Coffee, tea, or club soda with lemon or lime

TV SNACK
Popcorn (unsalted)

BEDTIME SNACK
Cup low-fat milk

SIXTH DAY

BREAKFAST
Orange juice
Poached egg
Whole-wheat toast with margarine
Coffee or tea

MORNING COFFEE BREAK
Approved snacks and soft drinks

LUNCH
Apple juice
Sliced turkey sandwich
Salad composed of raw turnip slices, pepper rings,
and dressing of your choice
Pickles and condiments (optional)
Orange sherbet (or other fruit sherbet)
Any approved soft drink

AFTERNOON COFFEE BREAK
Approved snacks and soft drinks

DINNER
Cocktail, hard liquor, beer, or wine (optional)
Beef stew composed of lean beef, potatoes, carrots,
and onions
Tomato salad with dressing of your choice
Slice whole-wheat bread
Pickles and condiments (optional)
Fresh fruit cup
Coffee, tea, or club soda with lemon or lime

TV SNACK
Cheese chunks with slice whole-wheat bread cut into
small pieces

BEDTIME SNACK
Cup low-fat milk

SEVENTH DAY

BREAKFAST
Half grapefruit
Farina
Low-fat milk
Toast with peanut butter

MORNING COFFEE BREAK
Approved snacks and soft drinks

LUNCH
Split-pea soup
Tossed green salad with blue-cheese dressing
Hard roll
Canned peaches (in light syrup)
Any approved soft drink

AFTERNOON COFFEE BREAK
Approved snacks and soft drinks

DINNER
Cocktail, hard liquor, beer, or wine (optional)
Roast chicken
Large baked potato
Baked squash
Coleslaw
Slice whole-wheat bread with margarine
Pickles and condiments (optional)
Coffee, tea, or club soda with lemon or lime

TV SNACK
  Popcorn (unsalted)

BEDTIME SNACK
  Cup low-fat milk

WHO WILL LOSE WEIGHT ON THE I LOVE NEW YORK EATING HOLIDAY

If you weigh more than 135 pounds at the start of the Eating Holiday, you'll continue to lose weight while enjoying seven delicious and filling meals each day. The heavier you are, the more weight you'll lose.

"It was the most beautiful experience of my life," a svelte prima donna, who once weighed 185 pounds, enthused. "I'd lost thirteen pounds the first week, and I would have been happy just to have held my weight steady for the second week, but I actually lost two more pounds! And I was having such a good time while I was doing it!"

If you weigh less than 135 pounds as you go into the second week, you'll hold your weight rock-steady during your Eating Holiday.

Any questions?

Yes. Isn't there a chance that after dieting a full week, I'll overeat on the first day of my Eating Holiday and gain weight?

You wouldn't be human if you didn't. But don't panic. The next day your body will rebel at the thought of excess food to the extent that you'll eat less than you would ordinarily, and·you'll lose the weight you gained. Bill knows; it happened to him. After that, you'll eat just as much as you need to feel satisfied.

I lost all the weight I wanted to lose during the first week. Do I have to go on an Eating Holiday?

You certainly do. You're not only losing weight during the first two weeks, you're also learning new food preferences and new eating habits that will help keep you slim for the rest of your life. You need the second week to reinforce what you learned the week before.

Should your scoreboard show you're continuing to lose more weight during the second week, just eat more. Since you're a food lover, that should be a delight. *Caution:* Don't go wild when you eat more. Watch your scale.

8

How to Lose *More* Weight Easily

You've LOST ABOUT ten pounds the first week. You've lost up to three pounds the second week, or kept your weight stable. Now you want to lose more weight.

It's simple.

You just go back to the I Love New York 7-Day Crash Program for another week.

At the end of that week, take another one-week I Love New York Eating Holiday.

If you still want to lose more weight return once again to the Crash Program and follow it with yet another Eating Holiday.

Continue on alternate Crash Programs and Eating Holidays until you're down to desired weight.

Remember to weigh yourself every day before breakfast and keep your appropriate scoreboard up to date.

(You'll find a supply of first- and second-week score-boards at the end of this book.)

What happens if I get down to desired weight before the end of a Crash Program week?

Start your final Eating Holiday the next day. Always end your reducing program with an Eating Holiday.

What happens if I get down to weight during an Eating Holiday?

Continue your Holiday to the end of the week, but to keep your weight steady, eat more.

CASE HISTORY: THIRTY-POUND WEIGHT LOSS IN THREE WEEKS

S. L. is a slim, debonair Wall Street executive. He wasn't always.

"My doctor insisted I lose thirty pounds," he told us. "My wife agreed with him. I had put on the weight fast—oh, maybe in two, three months. There was a death in the family and I lost a small fortune in futures, both around the same time. I suppose that's what triggered it off. I must have gorged myself to drown my sorrows. You know, I've read some place there's more foodaholics than there are alcoholics. I was hooked on food, and I didn't think I'd ever be able to slim down again.

"After the doctor and my wife, Susan, read the riot act to me, I decided to go on the I Love New York Diet. I never believed it would work. But did it work! I lost two pounds the first day, and I was so encouraged I was eager to stay on it. I'll admit that in a few days the compulsion to stuff myself returned—I'd had a pretty bad day at the office, it was raining, and I couldn't get a cab, and all sorts of things had gone wrong. But I said to myself, 'Don't panic. In just a few days you can go on an Eating Holiday and binge without feeling guilty.' So I stuck it out.

"Was I glad! At the end of the first week I had lost thirteen pounds! Now I was really motivated to go ahead and lose the other seventeen pounds.

"The second week—the week on the Eating Holiday— the pressure was off, and I was glad I had a chance to relax. There were lots of my favorite foods, and I ate until I was filled up at every meal—all seven of them. This was the week when I took out a snapshot of me taken just before I had begun to put on weight, and taped it on my full-length mirror right next to my scoreboard. I looked athletic and trim. I'm six five, and I remember when my wife took the shot she said, 'You should be playing Tarzan opposite Bo Derek.' *That* was what I wanted to look like again.

"Only fourteen pounds stood between me and looking like Tarzan again. I say *only* fourteen pounds, because now I was convinced I could get it off, and I thought I had a shot at getting it off in a week. I was confident, since by now I had two weeks of dieting experience under my belt—and I *mean* that as a pun—and I was used to eating low-fat food, and I had made all those hints on quicker weight loss a part of my life-style. I was exercising daily again—jogging for at least a half hour; I was cutting down on salt; I was eating very, v-e-r-y slowly; and I was calling it a meal the instant I felt filled up. I had all the big guns going for me. How could I lose? Nobody but *nobody* could have stopped me from continuing on the I Love New York Diet for just one more final week.

"It was *easy*. It was *soooooo* easy. I started on a Wednesday, and on Thursday morning of the next week I weighed myself before breakfast, and—I'd done it! I'd *really* done it—I'd taken off thirty pounds in just three weeks! I was down to my Tarzan weight. It was such a wonderful moment, I let out a Tarzan yell.

"And I felt like swinging from the treetops all during the final Eating Holiday week."

HEAVY-WEIGHT-LOSS PROGRAMS

If you're a big man or woman you can lose about thirty pounds in three to four weeks.

Week 1. Follow the 7-Day Crash Program
Week 2. Take an Eating Holiday.
Week 3. Repeat *Week 1.*
Week 4. Repeat *Week 2.*

You can lose even more weight by continuing to alternate the 7-Day Crash Program with the Eating Holiday.

On a six-week Program you can lose about forty-five pounds.

On an eight-week Program you can lose about sixty pounds.

You can lose as much weight as you want to lose—simply, steadily, and safely.

Getting down to your desired weight is one of the greatest personal accomplishments of your life. It's a red-letter day, as exciting as the day you buy your first house or make your first million. You're proud, excited, glowing with self-esteem. People are telling you, "My God, you did it! How youthful you've become! You're so slim!" You've done something that only a small—a *very* small—percentage of people are able to do. You have every right to feel ecstatic.

So imagine how you'll feel when you *keep it off permanently.*

Do it the easy way.

Just follow the instructions in the next chapter.

9

The I Love New York Lifetime Stay-Slim Program

How OFTEN HAVE YOU seen a dieter get down to ideal weight and the next day gorge on pizza and banana splits? If that dieter is you, you know your real problem is not taking it off, it's *keeping* it off.

Dr. Norman Jolliffe wrote: "Ninety percent of people who successfully reduce [on other diets] regain, sooner or later—more often sooner than later—their hard-lost weight." Some more recent estimates put the failure figure at 95 percent to 98 percent.

Dieters have perpetually wailed, "I lose weight, I gain it back, I lose weight, I gain it back.... I go on one diet after another, but the results are always the same. In a few months—a year at the most—I'm fatter than I was before. There must be some way, somehow, to stop the yo-yo effect."

There is.

According to Dr. Jolliffe, finding a way to break the yo-yo effect was a "unique purpose" of his weight-control program. That purpose was achieved by his Prudent Diet, one variation of which we call the I Love New York Lifetime Stay-Slim Program. During the period 1958 to 1972, only 5 percent of the Bureau of Nutrition's 1,100 volunteers regained any part of the lost weight. While other diets fail to keep it off, the Prudent Diet succeeds up to 30 percent of the time.

UNPARALLELED STAY-SLIM SUCCESS BASED ON WORLD-FAMOUS PSYCHOLOGICAL DISCOVERY

Dr. Jolliffe explains: "Habit is a very powerful factor in changing automatic bodily reflexes. In this connection [Dr. Ivan] Pavlov [a famous Russian physiologist] coined the expression 'conditioned reflex.' Using dogs, he would ring a bell and then promptly feed them. After keeping this up for some time he noted that if he rang the bell but did not feed them, the dogs would salivate *as if fed*. [That is, the dogs would react *automatically* to the sound of the bell.] This type of response is called a 'conditioned reflex.'"

Dr. Pavlov's psychological discovery, which created a sensation throughout the scientific world when it was announced, is the foundation for the Lifetime Stay-Slim

Program's success. Your "bell" is the time you sit down to your meal. When it's breakfast time, or lunch time, or dinner time, or any of the four snack times, you've been trained *by doing* to respond with a conditioned reflex—a new set of stay-slim eating habits. Your training came during your weeks on the 7-Day Crash Program and on the Eating Holidays.

As each meal "bell" rings, you mae the following *automatic* responses:

- You *eat* the meal. You never skip it.
- You eat only what's on the menu.
- You eat until you're just filled up. Then you stop.
- You eat slowly.
- You eat your salad *before* your main dish.
- You avoid commercial salad dressings.
- You prefer low-fat food.
- You trim away all fat from your meat, poultry, and fish.
- You prefer fish and vegetables cooked with little or no butter and salt.
- You prefer herbs and spices to salt.
- You never eat the skin of a chicken.
- You use margarine (preferably diet margarine) in small quantities instead of butter.
- You use pickles and other condiments sparingly.
- You prefer fresh food to canned or frozen food.
- You take your coffee or tea without sugar, cream, or whole milk.
- You prefer low-fat milk and cheese.
- You eat more fruit and vegetables than ever before.

And since the "bell" rings only at mealtime, *you do not eat between meals*—that deadly period when most good eating intentions give up the ghost.

WHAT TO EAT SPECIFICALLY TO STAY SLIM PERMANENTLY

Once you're down to your desired weight, the whole great, big, wonderful world of stay-slim, healthful food is open to you. Experts at the Bureau of Nutrition advise that your meals "can consist of . . . commonly available foods that are palatable and nutritionally adequate, meeting the specific nutrient requirements of family members. [These] requirements . . . are best met with a balanced diet of varied foods selected from each of the [following] basic food groups":

Fruit. Eat these high-vitamin-C fruits *daily:* oranges, grapefruit, tangerines, cantaloupes, strawberries, mangoes, papayas, as well as other fruits in season.

Vegetables. Eat these high-vitamin-A vegetables *at least three to four times a week:* spinach, collards, kale, turnip greens, broccoli, watercress, carrots, pumpkin, sweet potatoes, zucchini, and winter squash, as well as other vegetables.

Whole-grain and enriched breads, and whole-grain foods. "Enriched" means that most or all of the essential nutrients lost in processing have been restored. Eat one of the following grain foods *at each meal:* Bread or rolls made with whole-grain flour or enriched processed flour, pasta, rice, cereals, cornmeal, grits, and buckwheat. It's prudent to eat only three slices of bread, or one roll and two slices of bread, a day.

Eggs. Eat up to four *a week*—scrambled, sunny-side up, poached, boiled, prepared any way you like. You can even whip up an omelet, using approved ingredients. Just don't fry the eggs in butter. Use a non-stick skillet instead. If you like, you can add a very small amount of margarine ("diet" margarine preferred).

Milk. Drink two cups of low-fat or skim milk *daily*. You may substitute buttermilk, which, despite its name, is low in fat.

Fish, poultry, or lean meat. Eat two servings of two kinds of these high-protein foods *daily*. Have about equal servings of each of the three kinds *during the week*. Fish includes all kinds of shellfish, like crab, mussels, lobster, scallops, clams, shrimp, and oysters. Turkey and chicken are the preferred fowl. Lean meats include veal, beef, lamb, rabbit, venison, and fresh ham. Prepare all these foods with a minimum of salt and no rich sauces.

Oils. Consume one to two teaspoons of liquid vegetable oil *each day* in salads or in cooking. Acceptable oils are cottonseed, safflower, corn, soybean, or sunflower. Use margarine made predominantly from liquid vegetable oil.

NOT A DON'T-EAT
BUT A DO-EAT PROGRAM

In addition to the selections from the basic food groups, you can also enjoy the following favorites on your Lifetime Stay-Slim Program.

Alcoholic beverages. However, heed this advice:

—Stay away from sweetened cocktails, such as whiskey sours and old-fashioneds.

—If you like rum, be sure it's labeled dry (which means not sweet).

—Cokes and other soft drinks are fine as mixers, provided they contain no sugar.

—Dry wines are okay, but avoid dessert wines, such as French sauternes, port, sweet sherry, Marsala, and so on.

—Don't finish your meal with cordials or liqueurs; they're high in sugar.

—Low-calorie ("light") beer is preferred, but if you can't stand the taste (or rather the lack of it), a bottle of the real thing can't hurt you.

—Nothing wrong with rye, scotch, or Canadian whiskey, but bourbon is too sweet, and so is Irish whiskey. Irish coffee is even sweeter and is topped with whipped cream, a virtually all-fat no-no.

—Vodka and gin (alone or in a dry martini) get the stamp of approval, as do cognac and other brandies.

But this is not a "drinking man's" diet. Limit yourself to one glass of wine (about 4½ to 5 ounces), one jigger of hard liquor (about 1 to 1½ ounces), or one bottle or can of beer a day.

Hors d'oeuvres. "Low-calorie refreshments for conscientious weight reducers" is what nutrition specialists call the delectable tidbits created for you by the Bureau of Nutrition. For recipes, see Index.

Fruit juices. Apple, pineapple, orange, grapefruit, or any other, provided they're fresh or packed without sugar.

Mixed salads. Take garden-fresh salad greens, such as romaine, Bibb, and iceberg lettuce, chicory, escarole, and watercress, and combine them with your choice of onions, scallions, carrots, endives, radishes, tomatoes, cabbage, and celery—and you can toss salads as beautiful to look at as they are delicious to eat. You can eat as much as you like, using lemon and herb dressings, or oil and vinegar dressings, or dressings created specially for you by the Bureau of Nutrition. For recipes see Recipe Index.

Liver. You can substitute it for meat once or twice a month.

Beans, peas, and lentils (legumes), which are high in protein, can be used to supplement small portions of meat, fish, and poultry. They can also be combined with whole grains.

Cheese. One ounce of hard cheese may be substituted occasionally for two ounces of meat. Small quantities of cheese of any kind may be eaten as snacks; preferred varieties are cottage cheese, pot cheese, and farmer cheese.

Yogurt—provided it's the low-fat variety and contains no sugared additives.

Soup. Any that please your palate except creamed soups (try low-fat yogurt soups instead). Preferred are clear consommé, chicken broth, vegetable soup, and fish chowders. Chill soups to remove fat, then reheat before serving.

Desserts. You'll find recipes for mouth-watering confections prepared by the Bureau of Nutrition in the Recipe Index.

And for starchy-food lovers (and what former overweight isn't?), here are delectable—

Bread alternates. Instead of two slices of bread, you can have a bagel, or a pancake, or a muffin. Or you can replace your daily quota of three slices of bread (or two slices of bread and a hard roll) with three quarters cup of rice, mashed potatoes, noodles, spaghetti, or any other pasta. Instead of one slice of bread, try a small baked or boiled potato from time to time.

IT'S EASY TO MAKE UP YOUR OWN LIFETIME STAY-SLIM MENUS

"One of the great things about the 7-Day Crash Diet and the Eating Holiday," a slim, elegant clothes designer told us, "is that all the menus are laid out for you. I'm much too busy to be thinking about food. I wish the menus could be laid out for me for the rest of my life."

They are.

Not day by day, but as a general plan. All you have to do is fill in the specific foods you like best.

A SIMPLE LIFETIME MENU PLAN FOR PERMANENT SLIMNESS

BREAKFAST
Fruit
  High-vitamin-C fruit or fruit juice
Protein food (select one)
  Eggs, cheese, peanut butter, or fish
Whole-grain or enriched cereal
  Any commercial brand with low-fat milk
Bread
  Slice whole-wheat or enriched bread with margarine
Beverage
  Coffee, tea, or herb tea

MORNING COFFEE BREAK
Snack (select one)
  Almond macaroon, fruit, cottage cheese or pot cheese, plain low-fat yogurt
Beverage
  Coffee, tea, herb tea, or low-calorie soft drink

LUNCH
Fruit
  Bananas or any fruit of your choice

Salad
　　Any tossed salad with any approved dressing (see Recipe Index)
Vegetables
　　Any vegetable of your choice except potatoes
Protein food
　　Hot dish of fish, chicken, lean meat, or egg, with one slice bread or bread alternate (see page 80)
　　　　　　　　　　　or
　　Cold sandwich of fish, chicken, turkey, lean meat, egg, cheese, or peanut butter with soup of your choice except creamed soup
Dessert
　　Flavored gelatin (no sugar added), water ice, or sponge cake
Beverage
　　Coffee, tea, herb tea, low-fat milk, or buttermilk

AFTERNOON COFFEE BREAK
Snack (select one)
　　Fruit, nuts, open-faced peanut butter sandwich, plain low-fat yogurt
Beverage
　　Coffee, tea, herb tea, or low-calorie soft drink

DINNER
Predinner drink
　　Cocktail, hard liquor, beer, or wine (beer or wine may be enjoyed with the meal instead)
Hors d'oeuvres
　　For list of low-calorie delectables, see Chapter 16
　　　　　　　　　　　or

Fresh fruit cocktail

or

Seafood cocktail

Soup

Any of your choice except creamed soups

Salad

Any tossed salad with any approved dressing (see Recipe Index)

Vegetable

Potato, pasta, or any other bread alternate (see page 80), or vegetable of your choice

Protein food

Hot dish of fish, poultry, or lean meat

Bread

Whole-wheat or enriched-flour roll

Dessert

Angel food cake or sherbet

Beverage

Coffee, tea, or herb tea

TV SNACK

Snack (select one)

Raw carrots and celery, unsalted popcorn, peanut butter or hard-cheese cubes on bite-size slices of bread

Beverage

Low-calorie soft drink or beer (if not consumed during dinner)

BEDTIME SNACK (select one)

Whole-grain or enriched cereal with low-fat milk, or cup low-fat milk, or plain low-fat yogurt

Your meals can also include at your option: Jellies, jams, and preserves with non-caloric sweeteners; small amounts of mayonnaise as a spread; small amounts of margarine (diet margarine preferred) on bread and rolls, potatoes, and vegetables; unlimited quantities of herbs and spices for seasoning (example: pepper, paprika, and chives on potatoes); and a moderate amount of pickles and condiments.

YOU DON'T MISS THE NO-NO'S

The number one question a non-dieter asks a dieter is "What do you miss most?"

"The funny part is," a slender, attractive woman's editor of a national magazine said, "I don't miss anything. I'm conditioned not to. I once had a passion for chocolate ice cream, but you know something, it's not on the menus, so I didn't eat it for a couple of months, and then when I did, I had lost my taste for it!"

Staying with the diet conditions you to lose your taste for all fatty foods and for excessively salty ones as well.

A slim director of an art gallery who looks a great deal like a young Douglas Fairbanks, Jr., said, "You know I have some friends who put salt on salt. They douse everything with salt before they even taste it. I say, 'Why do you do that?' They say to me, 'Without salt, food is disgusting.' You know something? After just two weeks' conditioning to do without salt, I found food *with* salt disgusting."

You don't have to carry a long list of no-no's around with you. Because you're conditioned to eat only slimming foods, you *automatically* eliminate no-no's from your diet and develop an aversion to them.

10

How To Regain Your Slim Figure After You've Strayed

"IF YOU'RE CONDITIONED to stay on the I Love New York Stay-Slim Program," people ask, "how can you possibly stray?"

There are two ways, and neither of them is your fault.

Let's say, you're traveling, or there's a family crisis, or you're rushing to meet a deadline. You can't possibly sit down and eat at seven regular mealtimes. But those mealtimes are your conditioning "bell"; and when the bell doesn't ring, your conditioning breaks .down.

Or let's say, you're weekending with friends, or attending a convention, or vacationing, or spending the holidays with Grandma. You can arrange for the conditioning "bell" to ring at seven regular mealtimes, but the meals you're served won't consist of the I Love New York Diet slimming food. Without that correct response to the "bell," your conditioning breaks down.

In either case, by the time you've returned to your normal life-style, you've put on six to ten pounds—or more.

"When I look at myself in my full-length mirror after a long weekend, I could weep" is a familiar lament. "What's so terrible about it is I seem to have lost my stay-slim eating habits as well. I eat all the wrong foods, and I eat too much of them, and I *continue* to gain weight. How will I ever get my beautiful figure back again?"

Reinforce your conditioning, advised Dr. Norman Jolliffe, who discovered psychological conditioning as the basis of successful lifelong weight control. You can follow Dr. Jolliffe's advice with these

SEVEN SIMPLE STEPS TO REGAIN YOUR TRIM FIGURE

Step 1. Strip and weigh yourself before breakfast. Ugh!

Step 2. Study yourself carefully in your full-length mirror, full-face and profile, until you know the location of every bulge, bump, and blob of blubber. You're a mess. So do something about it *fast*.

Step 3. Tape an *I Love New York Diet Scoreboard* on your full-length mirror at eye level. (You'll find scoreboards at the end of this book.) Next to the scoreboard, tape a snapshot of yourself in a swimsuit, taken when you were still a 10. That's your goal.

Step 4. Go back on the I Love New York 7-Day Crash Program. You had fun on it before. You'll find it even more exciting this time. It's also easier because you've already gone through it at least once.

Step 5. Exercise daily. For the kinds of exercise that give the best results, see Chapter 14.

Step 6. At the end of the week or before, rejoice as your scoreboard shows you've lost all the weight you wanted to lose, and your full-length mirror reflects a figure as elegantly slim as the one in the snapshot.

Step 7. Celebrate by going on an I Love New York Eating Holiday.

In just two self-fulfilling weeks, you've regained your ideal weight and reinforced your conditioning. From now on under normal circumstances, you'll stay on the I Love New York Lifetime Stay-Slim Program, and keep your weight ideal, as automatically and effortlessly as you did before.

ARE YOU A VICTIM OF "CREEPING WEIGHT GAIN"?

"What's happened to me is very disturbing," a U.N. diplomat complained as we drove to Lincoln Center for the opening of the opera season. "I got down to my ideal weight, I went on the Stay-Slim Program, I did everything right, but over the course of four to six weeks, I put on a pound, and then another pound, and then another pound, and today I'm four pounds overweight. It's shocking. What's gone wrong?"

"You go to lots of parties?"

"But of course."

"How often does the hostess urge you to have just one more hors d'oeuvre?"

"Quite often."

"And how many times do you have more than one hors d'oeuvre?"

"As often as I'm asked. After all, I *am* a diplomat. But what possible difference can that make? How many calories does one little hors d'oeuvre have?"

Just a few. But many hors d'oeuvres over many days add up to a great many calories. The weight gain is slow: a small fraction of a pound, then another small fraction, then still another small fraction and so on. Most bathroom scales don't reflect fractional changes, so you're not aware of what's happening to you until your scale registers a sudden shocking extra pound, seemingly from out of the blue. That's creeping weight gain.

Creeping weight gain is one of the greatest dangers to anybody who desires to stay slim. It comes from eating that little extra portion of anything (except zero-calorie foods). If you add just one third slice of bread daily to each of your three major meals, you'll gain up to seven pounds a year. If you drink just one more jigger of scotch before dinner each night, your weight will increase one pound a month. If you nibble just a few salted peanuts between each of your seven meals every day, you'll gain a pound a week: Those tiny tastes of no-no's—dabs of mayonnaise, smidgens of ice cream, thin smears of butter—when repeated consistently can build into a fattening catastrophe.

If you've gained more than three pounds, and you can't explain how it happened, you may be a victim of creeping weight gain. Get that extra poundage off at once by taking the *Seven Simple Steps to Regain Your Trim Figure* (see page 88). Then use the following rules to put a stop to creeping weight gain before it begins. Even if you've escaped so far, it's wise to follow the rules. An ounce of prevention is worth a pound of fat.

HOW TO PREVENT CREEPING WEIGHT GAIN

· Don't make a habit of tasting foods not on your approved menus. Of course you can taste. A tenth of a teaspoon of even the most whipped-creamy, chocolate-syruped, triple-scoop ice cream extravaganza has less than ten calories. Just don't do it ten times or more a day every day. Allow yourself just two tastes of non-menu foods a day—no more. And remember, a taste is not a mouthful or more; it's a tenth of a teaspoon or less.

· *Don't overload your plate.* When there's more food on your plate than you need to feel filled up, there's the temptation to take an extra mouthful or two. Avoid that temptation by putting no more on your plate than experience tells you is enough to produce that filled-up feeling. For most of us, restaurant-sized portions are just about right.

• *Practice snack control.* The "I Love New York Diet snack law" states: If there's a snack within reach, you'll reach for it. So place within reach only enough snacks to fill you up. Snack control means weight control.

• *Never eat between meals.* Seven meals a day should be enough for anybody. Don't alibi with "Oh, I just nibble." One chronic nibbler was told by his psychologist to keep a record of what he nibbled and how much. At the end of one day, the total calories nibbled topped 2,000. On the Lifetime Stay-Slim Program, those extra calories could cause a horrendous gain of four pounds a week! I cite this unusual example as a warning. But even mild between-meal nibbling is a slimness destroyer.

There's one exception to the never-eat-between-meals rule. With mealtime an hour or so away, you could become genuinely hungry. Reasons include stress, prolonged exercise, sex, boredom, and hard work. To quell your between-meal hunger pangs, eat your fill of raw carrots, celery, turnips, radishes, cucumbers, and other raw vegetables. (You can keep them fresh and crunchy in your refrigerator in a covered container partially filled with cold water.) Very low in calories and extremely high in fiber, raw vegetables fill you up but don't fill you out.

• *Drink as much water as you like as often as you like.* With your stomach filled with this calorie-free liquid, you'll be less likely to nibble, overtaste, or reach for just one more of anything. Equally as effective as water are coffee, tea, and herb teas (no sugar, cream, or whole milk added to any of them), mineral water, and soft drinks that are virtually non-caloric. Carbonated beverages are particularly effective in giving you that filled-up feeling.

• *Keep your refrigerator and cupboards virtually bare.* You can't eat extras if they aren't around. Stock only enough edibles for one day's approved menus. One of New York's most glamorous show-biz personalities keeps in her refrigerator only the day's food requirements and a fresh rose.

"Why the rose?"

"It's a love token to myself for having the common sense to keep out all temptation."

"PSEUDO-SATISFACTION" AND WHAT YOU CAN DO ABOUT IT

"I eat all the right foods. I don't nibble between meals, gobble extras, or cheat. I eat only until I'm satisfied. But I gain weight on the Stay-Slim Program. What's wrong?"

That's a familiar question. The answer is always the same: You don't realize it but you're eating too fast.

Speed eating can put more weight on you per day than an extra pound of chocolates, three boxes of cookies, or a quart of ice cream. That's because when you eat fast, you don't feel satisfied until you've consumed more calories than your body needs. That's pseudo-satisfaction.

There's a scientific explanation for it. It takes X minutes (the number of minutes differs from person to person) for a just-enough meal to digest and enter the bloodstream. When it does, a trigger mechanism goes off in your body and your nervous system signals that you're satisfied. When you finish your meal in ½X minutes, there's no signal. You go on eating for X minutes, and by that time you've gobbled up two meals. Speed up your eating to ⅓X minutes, and you can eat three meals before the trigger mechanism goes off. The faster you eat, the more you take in before you're satisfied.

Slow eating is the key to slim eating. And the key to slow eating is chewing.

One of the most popular fortune cookie messages reads: "Every man eats, but Fu Manchu." It's true. Chewing is an art practiced mainly by the mandarins of our society, such as New York's beautiful people. Dining to them is an exquisite ritual. Relaxed, they chew with deliberate slowness to extract the subtle flavors of the food and experience taste sensations utterly unknown to fast eaters.

But chewing is only one way to slow down your eating speed. Here's—

THE COMPLETE
I LOVE NEW YORK DIET
SLOW-EATING GUIDE

• *Regard each cooked dish as a work of art.* (The I Love . New York Diet gourmet dishes are just as good to look at as they are to eat. Recipes begin on page 127.) Take a minute or so to enjoy the appearance of your food before you begin to eat. That sets a leisurely pace for the entire meal.

• *Use your table utensils to eat all food,* including fruit, sandwiches, bread, and rolls. That's slower than eating with your hands.

• *Cut your food into many small pieces.* That takes time. Eating many small pieces takes more time.

• *Bring your food to your mouth with a slow, graceful motion.* Don't shovel it in like a high-speed feeding machine.

• *Put only one kind of food in your mouth at a time.* Eating meat, bread, and vegetables separately takes three times as long as eating them together.

• *Take advantage of the secret of slow chewing: Don't swallow until you've extracted the last bit of taste.* Dr. Peter A. Wish, a clinical psychologist specializing in weight control, advises you to put down your eating utensils as soon as you begin to chew; then after swallowing, count up to ten slowly before picking them up again.

• *Sip, don't swig, your beverages.* Let them linger on your palate and enjoy their full flavor (yes, even diet soda) before you let them slide down your throat.

95

· *Refrain from eating from time to time to chat with your dining companions.* Mom's admonition, "Don't talk with your mouth full," makes sense.

· *Take time out between courses.* All gourmets do it because it makes the next course taste so much better.

Benefit from the Slow-Eating Guide not only on the Lifetime Stay-Slim Program, but also on the 7-Day Crash Program and the Eating Holiday.

One convert to slow eating raved, "I'm tasting flavors I never dreamed existed before. You couldn't buy them from the greatest chefs in the world, and here they are in my favorite foods!" She used to be pleasingly plump, and now she's teasingly trim. "And I'm going to stay that way for the rest of my life. I never thought staying slim could be so—*delicious.*"

11

The I Love New York Diet Guide to Eating Out Without Tears

"I'VE BEEN ON MOST diets, but—hurray!—this one *really* lets me eat out and enjoy it," a now-slim cosmetics executive confided. "My job keeps me eating out more than I eat in, but on this diet—wow!—no hassle, no fuss, and I don't have to carry a package of raw vegetables and sunflower seeds around with me all day. Look what I had for lunch today—mountains of steamed clams and a forest of crisp, luscious salad. And that was for starters! I eat what I like, and as much as I like, in all the restaurants I like. I *love* staying slim in restaurants!"

Thanks to the practical scientists who devised the sound diets on which ours is based, the I Love New York Diet can easily be adopted by people who have to eat at least five major meals (lunches) and ten minor meals (snacks) each week away from home. There is *nothing* on this "do-able" diet that you can't get in most restaurants. You can eat out on the 7-Day Crash Program, the Eating Holiday, and the Lifetime Stay-Slim Program— comfortably and deliciously.

When I (Bill) was dieting, I prepared carefully each time I ate out. Before leaving home, I referred to the I Love New York Diet menus, and wrote out my order for lunch, breakfast, or dinner. At the restaurant I handed my order to the waiter. I admit I begrudged the work I had to do and the time it took out of my life. You would have felt the same way. That's why I worked out for you—

THE INSTANT, EFFORTLESS WAY TO PLACE ORDERS FOR I LOVE NEW YORK DIET MEALS IN MOST RESTAURANTS

On the following pages you'll find sample orders for I Love New York 7-Day Crash Program meals and Eating Holiday meals. Each breakfast, lunch, and dinner order is labeled Day 1, Day 2, Day 3, and so on. There are additional Order Forms at the back of this book. Just clip out the appropriate order and hand it to the waiter. That's all there is to it.

Following the I Love New York Diet Restaurant Order Forms in this chapter, you'll find an I Love New York Diet Restaurant Lifetime Stay-Slim Wallet Card. This is your guide to eating out without weight gain for the rest of your life.

THE I LOVE NEW YORK
7-DAY CRASH DIET
RESTAURANT ORDER FORMS

BREAKFAST MENUS

DAY 1: BREAKFAST   THE I LOVE NEW YORK
                              7-DAY CRASH DIET

Orange
Egg, boiled or poached
Piece Melba toast
Coffee or tea

DAY 2: BREAKFAST   THE I LOVE NEW YORK
                              7-DAY CRASH DIET

Grapefruit
Cottage cheese (or low-fat pot cheese)
Coffee or tea

DAY 3: BREAKFAST THE I LOVE NEW YORK
7-DAY CRASH DIET

Orange
Puffed wheat (preferably with no salt added)
Low-fat milk
Coffee or tea

DAY 4: BREAKFAST THE I LOVE NEW YORK
7-DAY CRASH DIET

Grapefruit
Shredded wheat
Low-fat milk
Coffee or tea

DAY 5: BREAKFAST THE I LOVE NEW YORK
7-DAY CRASH DIET

Tangerine or orange
½ thin-slice bread
Low-fat milk
Coffee or tea

DAY 6: BREAKFAST THE I LOVE NEW YORK
7-DAY CRASH DIET

Grapefruit
Egg, boiled or poached
Piece RyKrisp
Coffee or tea

DAY 7: BREAKFAST THE I LOVE NEW YORK
7-DAY CRASH DIET

Orange
Shredded wheat
Low-fat milk
Coffee or tea

LUNCH MENUS

DAY 1: LUNCH   THE I LOVE NEW YORK
                     7-DAY CRASH DIET

Shrimp or seafood of your choice
Celery, lettuce, tomatoes, and carrot sticks
Coffee, tea, or diet soda

DAY 2: LUNCH   THE I LOVE NEW YORK
                     7-DAY CRASH DIET

Sliced roast beef
Lettuce, celery, and tomatoes
Coffee, tea, or diet soda

DAY 3: LUNCH   THE I LOVE NEW YORK
                     7-DAY CRASH DIET

Fresh fruit salad
Cottage cheese
Coffee, tea, or diet soda

DAY 4: LUNCH   THE I LOVE NEW YORK
7-DAY CRASH DIET

Canned fish, such as tuna (oil removed, or packed in water or
*   broth)*
Lettuce, cucumbers, celery, and radishes
Coffee, tea, or club soda with lemon or lime

DAY 5: LUNCH   THE I LOVE NEW YORK
7-DAY CRASH DIET

Broiled hamburger
Green salad with sliced tomatoes
Coffee, tea, or diet soda

DAY 6: LUNCH   THE I LOVE NEW YORK
7-DAY CRASH DIET

Chicken or turkey slices
Lettuce, celery, and tomatoes
Coffee, tea, or diet soda

DAY 7: LUNCH   THE I LOVE NEW YORK
7-DAY CRASH DIET

Sliced hard-cooked eggs
Mixed green salad
Coffee, tea, or diet soda

DINNER MENUS

DAY 1: DINNER THE I LOVE NEW YORK
7-DAY CRASH DIET

Fresh fruit cocktail
Sautéed chicken breasts
Cabbage, turnips, and zucchini (or Brussels sprouts)
Coffee, tea, or club soda with lemon or lime

DAY 2: DINNER THE I LOVE NEW YORK
7-DAY CRASH DIET

Tomato juice or V-8 (preferably with no salt added)
Broiled liver
Spinach, cauliflower, celery, and green pepper
Coffee, tea, or club soda with lemon or lime

DAY 3: DINNER THE I LOVE NEW YORK
7-DAY CRASH DIET

Clams
Flounder, haddock, or fish of your choice
Celery, radishes, carrots, and zucchini (or cabbage)
Coffee, tea, or club soda with lemon or lime

DAY 4: DINNER   THE I LOVE NEW YORK
7-DAY CRASH DIET

Roast veal
Mixed green salad
Strawberries or other berries in season
Coffee, tea, or club soda with lemon or lime

DAY 5: DINNER   THE I LOVE NEW YORK
7-DAY CRASH DIET

Broiled chicken
Asparagus, spinach, and cauliflower
Fresh fruit salad
Coffee, tea, or club soda with lemon or lime

DAY 6: DINNER   THE I LOVE NEW YORK
7-DAY CRASH DIET

Steak or London broil
Broccoli, string beans, and green peppers
Strawberries
Coffee, tea, or club soda with lemon or lime

DAY 7: DINNER   THE I LOVE NEW YORK
7-DAY CRASH DIET

Crabmeat or seafood of your choice
Spinach, broccoli, and carrots
Grapefruit
Coffee, tea, or club soda with lemon or lime

THE I LOVE NEW YORK EATING HOLIDAY RESTAURANT ORDER FORMS

BREAKFAST MENUS

DAY 1: BREAKFAST THE I LOVE NEW YORK EATING HOLIDAY

Pineapple juice
Slice whole-wheat toast with margarine (diet margarine preferred)
Cream of wheat
Low-fat milk
Raisins
Coffee or tea

DAY 2: BREAKFAST THE I LOVE NEW YORK EATING HOLIDAY

Orange
Canadian bacon
Slice toast with margarine (diet margarine preferred)
Coffee or tea

DAY 3: BREAKFAST   THE I LOVE NEW YORK EATING HOLIDAY

Orange
Hot oatmeal
Low-fat milk
Coffee or tea

DAY 4: BREAKFAST   THE I LOVE NEW YORK EATING HOLIDAY

Grapefruit juice
Wheat flakes
Low-fat milk
Swiss cheese
Slice toast
Coffee or tea

DAY 5: BREAKFAST   THE I LOVE NEW YORK EATING HOLIDAY

Blend of orange and grapefruit juice
Any ready-to-eat breakfast cereal
Low-fat milk
Slice toast with margarine (diet margarine preferred)
Coffee or tea

DAY 6: BREAKFAST   THE I LOVE NEW YORK
EATING HOLIDAY

Orange juice
Poached egg
Whole-wheat toast with margarine (diet margarine preferred)
Coffee or tea

DAY 7: BREAKFAST   THE I LOVE NEW YORK
EATING HOLIDAY

Half grapefruit
Farina
Low-fat milk
Toast with peanut butter

LUNCH MENUS

DAY 1: LUNCH   THE I LOVE NEW YORK EATING HOLIDAY

Grapefruit juice
Canned mackerel
Mixed green salad and dressing of your choice
Bread
Pickles and condiments (optional)
Any approved soft drink

DAY 2: LUNCH   THE I LOVE NEW YORK EATING HOLIDAY

Tomato juice
Chef's salad, composed of hard-cooked eggs, lean ham, chicken, and dressing of your choice
Pickles and condiments (optional)
Sponge cake
Any approved soft drink

DAY 3: LUNCH **THE I LOVE NEW YORK EATING HOLIDAY**

Tomato juice
Lean sliced beef
Lettuce wedges with salad dressing of your choice
Slice rye bread with margarine (diet margarine preferred)
Pickles and condiments (optional)
Angel food cake
Any approved soft drink

DAY 4: LUNCH **THE I LOVE NEW YORK EATING HOLIDAY**

Tomato juice
Chopped liver
2 slices rye bread
Cucumbers and radishes

Pickles and condiments (optional)
Baked apple
Any approved soft drink

DAY 5: LUNCH **THE I LOVE NEW YORK EATING HOLIDAY**

Tuna salad with dressing of your choice
Mixed raw vegetables
Slice whole-wheat bread with margarine (diet margarine preferred)
Pickles and condiments (optional)
Sherbet
Any approved soft drink

DAY 6: LUNCH THE I LOVE NEW YORK EATING HOLIDAY

Apple juice
Sliced turkey sandwich
Salad composed of raw turnip slices, pepper rings, and dressing of your choice
Pickles and condiments (optional)
Orange sherbet (or other fruit sherbet)
Any approved soft drink

DAY 7: LUNCH THE I LOVE NEW YORK EATING HOLIDAY

Split-pea soup
Tossed green salad with blue-cheese dressing
Hard roll
Canned peaches (in light syrup)
Any approved soft drink

DINNER MENUS

DAY 1: DINNER   THE I LOVE NEW YORK
                      EATING HOLIDAY

Cocktail, hard liquor, beer, or wine (optional)
Chicken with noodles
Green peas
Eggplant salad
Whole-grain bread
Pickles and condiments (optional)
Melon (if not in season, any other fresh fruit)
Coffee, tea, or club soda with lemon or lime

DAY 2: DINNER   THE I LOVE NEW YORK
                      EATING HOLIDAY

Cocktail, hard liquor, beer, or wine (optional)
Baked fish
Salad composed of pasta shells, cooked greens, and dressing of
*   your choice*
Fresh fruit cup
Coffee, tea, or club soda with lemon or lime

DAY 3: DINNER   THE I LOVE NEW YORK EATING HOLIDAY

Cocktail, hard liquor, beer, or wine (optional)
Broiled fish
Potato salad
Cooked greens
Corn bread with margarine (diet margarine preferred)
Coffee, tea, or club soda with lemon or lime

DAY 4: DINNER   THE I LOVE NEW YORK EATING HOLIDAY

Cocktail, hard liquor, beer, or wine (optional)
Lean pork with bean sprouts
Brown rice
Spinach
Hard roll
Pickles and condiments (optional)
Pineapple cubes (fresh or packed in own juices)
Coffee, tea, or club soda with lemon or lime

DAY 5: DINNER THE I LOVE NEW YORK
EATING HOLIDAY

Cocktail, hard liquor, beer, or wine (optional)
Red beans and rice
Tomato salad with dressing of your choice
Slice bread with margarine (diet margarine preferred)
Fresh fruit cup
Coffee, tea, or club soda with lemon or lime

DAY 6: DINNER THE I LOVE NEW YORK
EATING HOLIDAY

Cocktail, hard liquor, beer, or wine (optional)
Beef stew composed of lean beef, potatoes, carrots, and onions
Tomato salad with dressing of your choice
Slice whole-wheat bread
Pickles and condiments (optional)
Fresh fruit cup
Coffee, tea, or club soda with lemon or lime

DAY 7: DINNER   THE I LOVE NEW YORK
EATING HOLIDAY

Cocktail, hard liquor, beer, or wine (optional)
Roast chicken
Large baked potato
Baked squash
Cole slaw
Slice whole-wheat bread with margarine (diet margarine preferred)
Pickles and condiments (optional)
Coffee, tea, or club soda with lemon or lime

THE I LOVE NEW YORK
LIFETIME STAY-SLIM WALLET CARD

The Bureau of Nutrition, New York City Department of Health, makes this estimate of its Prudent Diet on which much of our maintenance diet is based: "It is designed to meet the nutrient needs of the family... and control weight for those who have maintained or achieved desirable weight. Tasty and nutritious, you can follow [it] and enjoy it... in restaurants."

But in a restaurant you don't have the time to study the general Simple Lifetime Menu Plan for permanent Slimness (page 81) and make specific choices. Instead choose swiftly from the approved foods listed on this Lifetime Stay-Slim Wallet Card. A permanent record of your Stay-Slim Restaurant Choices appears on p. 119.

DETACH AND CARRY IN YOUR WALLET

THE I LOVE NEW YORK DIET STAY-SLIM RESTAURANT CHOICES

Breakfast

Fresh fruit in season
Fresh fruit juices (or processed juices with no sugar added)
Hot or cold cereals with low-fat milk
Broiled kippers on toast
Canadian bacon
Toast or breakfast rolls with margarine

Lunch

Sandwiches (no butter or mayonnaise):
Fish, chicken, or turkey salad
Sliced chicken, turkey, lean ham, or sliced egg
Smoked salmon
Canadian bacon
Peanut butter

or

Salad platters:
Chicken or turkey salad plate
Cottage cheese and fresh fruit
Individual small can of tuna or salmon

NOTE: All salad platters may be served with your choice of lettuce, tomatoes, potato salad, coleslaw, green peppers, and other vegetables, plus two slices of bread or a hard roll. Oil and vinegar dressing are preferred.

or

Soup:
Any clear soup with two slices of bread or a hard roll

NOTE: You may substitute any approved sandwich for the bread or hard roll.

Dinner

Alcoholic beverage:
Any of your choice if desired

Appetizers:
Half grapefruit (with non-caloric sweetener)
Fresh fruit cup
Tomato juice (preferably with no salt added)
Seafood cocktail (sauce on the side)
Pickled herring (without sour cream)

Salad:
Tossed salad of your choice, oil and vinegar dressing

Soup:
Any clear soup

Vegetables:
Baked or boiled white potato, sweet potato or yams (without butter or sour cream; a small amount of margarine is permissible)
Choice of green or yellow vegetable

Entrées:
Broiled or baked fish or seafood

Broiled or roast chicken or turkey (Cornish game hen is also permissible)
Broiled or roast veal
Roast leg of lamb
London broil or sirloin steak
Broiled or baked ham

Desserts:
Fresh fruit in season or processed fruit with no sugar added
Sherbet or ices
Flavored gelatin (no whipped cream)
Angel food or sponge cake
Plain yogurt

NOTE: You may include any of these desserts on your luncheon menu.

All Meals

Pickles and condiments:
Any in moderation

Beverages:
Coffee or tea (with non-caloric sweetener, and without whole milk or cream)
Low-fat milk
Buttermilk
Low-calorie sodas
Mineral water
Water
Fruit juices (with no added sugar)

THE I LOVE NEW YORK DIET
STAY-SLIM RESTAURANT CHOICES

Breakfast

Fresh fruit in season

Fresh fruit juices (or processed juices with no sugar added)

Hot or cold cereals with low-fat milk

Broiled kippers on toast

Canadian bacon

Toast or breakfast rolls with margarine

Lunch

Sandwiches (no butter or mayonnaise):

Fish, chicken, or turkey salad

Sliced chicken, turkey, lean ham, or sliced egg

Smoked salmon

Canadian bacon

Peanut butter

or

Salad platters:

Chicken or turkey salad plate

Cottage cheese and fresh fruit

Individual small can of tuna or salmon

NOTE: All salad platters may be served with your choice of lettuce, tomatoes, potato salad, coleslaw, green peppers, and other vegetables, plus two slices of bread or a hard roll. Oil and vinegar dressing are preferred.

or

Soup:

Any clear soup with two slices of bread or a hard roll

NOTE: You may substitute any approved sandwich for the bread or hard roll.

Dinner

Alcoholic beverage:

Any of your choice if desired

Appetizers:

Half grapefruit (with non-caloric sweetener)

Fresh fruit cup

Tomato juice (preferably with no salt added)

Seafood cocktail (sauce on the side)

Pickled herring (without sour cream)

Salad:

Tossed salad of your choice, oil and vinegar dressing

Soup:

Any clear soup

Vegetables:

Baked or boiled white potato, sweet potato or yams (without butter or sour cream; a

small amount of margarine
is permissible)
Choice of green or yellow
vegetable

Entrées:
Broiled or baked fish or sea-
food
Broiled or roast chicken or
turkey (Cornish game hen
is also permissible)
Broiled or roast veal
Roast leg of lamb
London broil or sirloin steak
Broiled or baked ham

Desserts:
Fresh fruit in season or
processed fruit with no
sugar added
Sherbet or ices
Flavored gelatin (no whipped
cream)

Angel food or sponge cake
Plain yogurt

NOTE: You may include any of
these desserts on your luncheon menu.

All Meals

Pickles and condiments:
Any in moderation

Beverages:
Coffee or tea (with non-caloric
sweetener, and without
whole milk or cream)
Low-fat milk
Buttermilk
Low-calorie sodas
Mineral water
Water
Fruit juices (with no added
sugar)

12

Answers to Your Questions About Eating Out While Slimming Down and Staying Slim

Many restaurant entrées come with a sauce. Okay to eat?

No. Restaurant sauces are too fat and salty. Request that the sauce be served on the side. Then just taste it and ask the waiter to take it away. Better still, instruct the waiter, "No sauce, please."

How about salad dressings?

Too many restaurants drench their salads with dressings heavy in fat, salt, and sugar. Ask instead for oil and vinegar.

When I order steak in a restaurant, it always comes with a layer of fat. What shall I do?

The same as you would do at home. Trim it off. Then ask your waiter to take it away. Leaving it on your plate may be an irresistible temptation.

My favorite restaurant places a basket of assorted rolls and breads on the table as soon as I sit down. How can I resist it?

Easily. Take one roll or the amount of bread the diet calls for, and ask the waiter to remove the rest. The restaurant bread basket is as dangerous as a hand grenade. Both can blow you up fast.

There are French-fried potatoes, home-fried potatoes, mashed potatoes—dozens of different kinds of potatoes. What kind shall I order?

Baked or boiled with no butter or sour cream. A moderate amount of margarine is permissible; and make that diet margarine if you're losing weight. Add all the chives the restaurant serves.

May I use salt and pepper?

Pepper, yes, to taste. Salt in moderation. Most gourmets don't ever touch the salt shaker. They prefer the natural taste of their food.

In the restaurants I go to, all the vegetables are cooked in butter. Is it all right to eat them?

No, it's not. Order a large salad instead.

How shall I order fish?

Broiled or baked with no butter, margarine, or oil, and light on the salt. Never order fish (or any food) fried.

Do I specifically ask the waiter for margarine instead of butter?

Yes, one pat. And ask for diet margarine while you're reducing. If none is available, skip margarine altogether.

How about ketchup?

Okay in moderation. Same advice for all other condiments and pickles.

Is cocktail sauce okay for my seafood cocktail?

Order the sauce on the side and use it in moderation. It's extremely high in sugar and salt. Try squeezing lemon juice over your cocktail instead. It perks up the natural flavors of the seafood, while cocktail sauce masks them.

How can I enjoy a broiled lobster without melted butter?

The same way you can enjoy a seafood cocktail without cocktail sauce. Squeeze lemon juice over the meat. Instead of tasting butter, you'll taste the true lobster flavor. Many gourmets never eat lobster any other way.

I have a special problem. I can't resist reading the menu. When I see apple pie, ice cream, and all the other mind-blowing desserts, the temptation is awful. What can I do?

If you're on the 7-Day Crash Program or the Eating Holiday, just hand in your Order Form and *don't* look at the menu. If you're on the Lifetime Stay-Slim Program, refer to your Wallet Card and *not* to the menu. (There's a way you *can* eat apple pie, ice cream, etc., and still stay slim. The secret is revealed on page 177. It's another wonder of the I Love New York Diet.)

There's nothing against having my bread toasted, is there?

Nothing at all. But don't think you're cutting down on calories that way. A slice of toast has as many calories as a slice of untoasted bread.

The I Love New York Diet doesn't mention English muffins. I love them. Can I substitute them for bread or rolls?

Not during the reducing weeks. Any substitution will weaken your conditioning. But life after dieting wouldn't be the same for you without all those delicious margarine-filled (not butter-filled) nooks and crannies. On the Lifetime Stay-Slim Program, enjoy!

What shall I do when a restaurant doesn't have something called for by the approved menu?

The same thing you would do when a restaurant is out of any food you order: Settle for a related food. If the waiter says, "No cauliflower," for example, order any other high-fiber food. (See page 195 for a selection.)

Almost all restaurant entrées are prepared with lots of fat and salt. How is it possible for me to eat them and diet?

It's not. Make certain your dishes are cooked to order and specify that they be prepared without fat. If the waiter rants, "Impossible!" tell him to have the chef use liquid vegetable oil instead. I've never known a chef to refuse. Always add these instructions to the waiter, "And tell the chef to go easy on the salt. Use herbs instead."

My favorite health-food restaurant serves maté. Does it get the green light?

Not during the reducing weeks. No substitutes are allowed. But if you've acquired a taste for maté, there's no reason why you shouldn't drink it after you've been conditioned. Maté is an herb tea that lifts your spirits, fights fatigue, and suppresses your appetite. You can also brew it at home.

Am I better off in a health-food restaurant than in a regular restaurant?

Not really. Most dishes in a health-food restaurant are as fat as or fattier than dishes in a regular restaurant and just as salty.

I love Chinese and Japanese food. On the Lifetime Stay-Slim Program can I indulge myself occasionally?

Once every two or three months. Oriental food is low in calories but high in sugar and salt. You won't gain fat tissue from a Chinese or Japanese meal, but you will gain water weight. Go back to the Stay-Slim Program at once, and the excess water will drain away.

I find restaurant eating an excuse for a binge. I'm out, it's costing me a bundle, so what-the-hell, why shouldn't I let myself go?

Before you let yourself go, think what you'll have to face in the mirror afterward: a bloated face, a bulging waistline, bags under your eyes, and that oh-why-did-I-do-it? expression. If you think just one costly restaurant meal is worth it, go ahead.

13

Stay-Slim Gourmet Recipes: Low-Calorie Versions of Favorite Dishes From All Over the World

DURING THE I LOVE NEW YORK DIET reducing weeks, you enjoy the same variety of foods you've been fond of all your life. When you're shedding weight, you don't want to be bothered with new and unfamiliar stints in the kitchen. Enjoying old favorites makes dieting so much easier.

But once down to your desired weight, with a lifetime ahead of you, you're eager to enjoy new adventures in eating. That's why the nutritionist-chefs at the Bureau of Nutrition, New York City Department of Health, concocted mouth-watering stay-slim dishes to satisfy even the most demanding gourmet. They're quick and easy to make, and so taste-packed they'll overcome any lingering desire you may have to backslide or binge.

One of the glories of these stay-slim recipes is that they're a sampling of the great cuisines of the world—

low-calorie versions of the dishes featured in New York's finest French, Italian, Oriental, Balkan, Hungarian, Near Eastern, Jewish, Puerto Rican, and other ethnic restaurants as well as in the best American restaurants. The kinds of food visitors flock to New York to enjoy at high prices are now available in your own home inexpensively—and without the excess calories.

"I've had my cook switch to these recipes, which pleases her because they're so easy," said a women's fashion sales director. After "a lifetime of attempts to lose weight on other diets,"—she had blitzed off thirty pounds on the I Love New York Diet and kept it off—"I simply couldn't keep it off before. So I tried dressing for slimness, making up for slimness, even took posture exercises to make me *appear* slim—but who was I kidding? Now I've stayed so slim—I'm 117 at five foot six—that I appear in my firm's commercials! Those aren't recipes. They're magic formulas for staying slim."

But you don't need to hire a cook to make them. "They were created to be used even by a novice cook," asserts Francine Prince, one of the nation's leading authorities on cooking for better health. "They're a marvelously simple way to get acquainted with the joys of healthful, slimming cooking." You'll have fun cooking these recipes, and you'll have more fun serving them to your guests. The dishes are so delicious your guests will never know they're eating low-calorie food.

Here are the I Love New York Stay-Slim Gourmet Recipes arranged alphabetically by the country of their origin. A recipe index at the end of the book will guide you to specific hors d'oeuvres, soups, entrées, and so on. Start today to cook your way to permanent slimness.

YOUR GUIDE TO I LOVE NEW YORK STAY-SLIM INTERNATIONAL RECIPES

AMERICAN RECIPES

COTTAGE CHEESE DIP

1½   *cups cottage cheese*
1   *tablespoon low-fat milk*
½   *teaspoon finely minced onion*
1   *tablespoon lemon juice*

Mix together. Serve with crisp vegetable dippers and thin crackers. *Yield:* About 1½ cups.

GARDEN HERB DIP

1   *recipe Cottage Cheese Dip*
¼   *teaspoon marjoram, or*
1   *teaspoon minced parsley*

Mix together. Serve with crisp vegetable dippers and thin crackers. *Yield:* About 1½ cups.

SPICY SEED DIP

1   *recipe Cottage Cheese Dip*
1   *teaspoon celery seed or caraway seed*

Mix together. Serve with crisp vegetable dippers and thin crackers. *Yield:* About 1½ cups.

CHIVE DIP

1 recipe Cottage Cheese Dip
2 tablespoons chopped chives

Mix together. Serve with crisp vegetable dippers and thin crackers. *Yield:* About 1½ cups.

CHILI DIP

1 recipe Cottage Cheese Dip
2 tablespoons chili sauce

Mix together. Serve with crisp vegetable dippers and thin crackers. *Yield:* About 1½ cups.

SEAFOOD DIP

1   recipe Cottage Cheese Dip
½ cup canned minced clams, drained well
    mashed sardines, tuna, or mackerel (all canned)
        to taste

Mix together. Serve with crisp vegetable dippers and thin crackers. *Yield:* About 2 cups.

COTTAGE CHEESE SALAD DRESSING

8 *ounces cottage cheese*
1/4 *cup cider vinegar*
3/4 *cup buttermilk*
1 *teaspoon oregano*
1/2 *teaspoon garlic powder*
1 *teaspoon salt*
1 *teaspoon sugar*
2 *stalks scallions, chopped fine*

In blender, whip cheese until liquid. Remove and place in bowl. Add remaining ingredients. Mix well. Chill before serving. *Serving suggestion:* Delicious with fruit, vegetable, and seafood salads. *Yield:* About 1¾ cups.

TARTAR SAUCE

1 *cup mayonnaise (page 146)*
1 *tablespoon finely chopped onion*
2 *tablespoons chopped dill pickles*
2 *tablespoons chopped parsley*
1 *tablespoon stuffed olives*

Mix all ingredients together. *Serving suggestion:* Sparks up broiled or baked fish or seafood. *Yield:* 1 cup.

TOMATO SAUCE

- 1   *onion, chopped*
- 1   *clove garlic, crushed (optional)*
- 4   *tablespoons vegetable oil*
- 1   *No. 2 can tomatoes*
- 1   *bay leaf or sprig sweet basil*
- ½   *teaspoon sugar*
- *salt and pepper to taste*

Sauté onion and garlic in oil for about 5 minutes. Add tomatoes, bay leaf or basil, and cook to a thick sauce (approximately ¾ hour). Add remainder of ingredients. Simmer 15 minutes. *Serving suggestion:* Adds flavor to meat loaf, fish, zucchini, eggplant, green peppers, spaghetti, rice, or noodles. *Yield:* 2 cups.

NEW ENGLAND FISH CHOWDER

- 1   *cup water*
- ½   *teaspoon salt*
- 1   *dash pepper*
- 1   *pound cod, haddock, whiting, or halibut*
- 2   *tablespoons vegetable oil*
- ½   *cup chopped onion*
- 1½   *cups diced raw potatoes*
- 1   *cup low-fat liquid milk, warmed*
- *chopped parsley or paprika*

Boil water. Add salt, pepper, and fish. Simmer 15 to 20 minutes. Do not boil. Remove bones and skin. Flake fish. Strain stock. In a pot, heat oil and add onion. Cook until transparent. Add fish stock and potatoes. Boil 15 minutes or until potatoes are done. Add milk and flaked fish. Simmer 2 or 3 minutes. Let stand several minutes to blend flavors before serving. Garnish with chopped parsley or paprika. *Yield:* Serves 4.

SAUTÉED MIXED VEGETABLES

1 *pound assorted leafy green vegetables (choose from broccoli rabe, chicory, escarole, mustard greens, and spinach)*
2 *tablespoons vegetable oil*
1 *clove garlic, crushed (optional)*
½ *teaspoon salt*

Remove roots and tough stalks. Wash thoroughly. Drain well. Heat oil in skillet or pan. Add garlic and brown. Add vegetables and salt. Sauté for 3 to 5 minues. *Yield:* Serves 4.

ASPARAGUS SAUTÉ

1 *pound asparagus*
2 *tablespoons vegetable oil*
1 *clove garlic, crushed (optional)*
½ *teaspoon salt*

Wash asparagus and cut stalks diagonally into 1-inch sections. Follow instructions for Sautéed Mixed Vegetables (preceding recipe). *Yield:* Serves 4.

PAN-FRIED FISH

1½ pounds fish (fillets, fish steak, or whole fish)
      salt and pepper to taste
   1 tablespoon lemon juice
      flour or cornmeal
   4 tablespoons vegetable oil

Season fish with salt and pepper. Sprinkle with lemon juice. Dip fish lightly in flour or cornmeal. Heat oil in skillet. Cook fish until golden brown on both sides (about 10 minutes). Serve with tartar sauce, tomato sauce, or mayonnaise (pages 132, 133, and 146, respectively) if desired. *Yield:* Serves 4.

BAKED FISH

   2 medium onions
   4 tablespoons vegetable oil
   1 No. 2 can tomatoes
   1 clove garlic, crushed
  ¼ teaspoon paprika
   1 teaspoon salt
      juice ½ lemon
   1 whole fish, about 2 pounds

Cut onions into thin slices and sauté in 2 tablespoons oil until golden brown. Add tomatoes, garlic, paprika, salt, lemon juice, and remaining oil. Simmer for about 20 minutes. Place fish in baking dish and cover with sauce. Bake in preheated oven at 350° for approximately 30 minutes. Remove from oven, garnish with parsley and lemon slices, and serve. *Yield:* Serves 4.

BROILED FISH

1½ *pounds fish (whole flat fish, split fish, steak, or fillets)*
    salt and pepper
    vegetable oil
    flour
    lemon juice, wine, or French Dressing (page 147) for basting

Season with salt and pepper. Brush with oil. Dust lightly with flour. Broil on well-oiled rack or aluminum foil for 5 to 10 minutes, depending on thickness of fish. Turn and broil 3 to 5 minutes more. Baste twice during broiling. *Yield:* Serves 4.

OVEN-FRIED CHICKEN

¼ *cup lemon juice*
¼ *cup vegetable oil*
¼ *teaspoon salt*
⅛ *teaspoon pepper*
¼ *teaspoon powdered thyme*
1 *frying chicken, cut into serving-size pieces*

To make marinade, combine lemon juice, oil, and seasonings. Pour over chicken parts, covering completely. Let stand in refrigerator for at least 1 hour. Bake, skin side down, in 350° oven for 25 to 30 minutes. Turn chicken skin side up and bake another 15 minutes or until done. *Yield:* Serves 4.

MEAT LOAF

$^1/_2$ cup bread crumbs or mashed potatoes
 1   medium onion, finely chopped
 1   teaspoon salt
$^1/_2$ teaspoon pepper
$^1/_2$ teaspoon marjoram
 2   eggs
$^1/_2$ cup cold broth (a dissolved bouillon cube may be used)
$^3/_4$ pound ground round or other lean beef
$^3/_4$ pound ground veal

Mix bread crumbs (or mashed potatoes), onion, salt, pepper, and marjoram. Beat eggs and mix with cold broth. Add all ingredients to meat and mix lightly with fork until well blended. Shape into an oblong loaf. Place in greased loaf pan (vegetable oil preferred) and bake in 350° oven for 45 to 60 minutes. *Yield:* Serves 5 to 6.

ORANGE MILK SHERBET

1   *cup evaporated skim milk*
1   *tablespoon lemon or lime juice*
1   *6-ounce can frozen orange juice concentrate (unsweetened)*
1   *tablespoon brandy, rum or liqueur (optional)*

Whip chilled milk until stiff (see *Note*). Fold in lemon juice. Gently mix in frozen concentrate. Add liquor. Freeze at once in prechilled freezer trays. *Yield:* 8 ½-cup portions.

Note: How to whip evaporated milk. Pour undiluted milk into freezer tray or directly into bowl for whipping. Chill in freezer compartment until fine crystals begin to form around the edges. Pour into cold bowl and whip rapidly with chilled beater until very stiff. When instructions are followed, evaporated milk will whip as stiffly as cream. If milk does not whip well, it is not cold enough. Just rechill and whip again.

PINEAPPLE MILK SHERBERT

1   *6-ounce can frozen pineapple juice concentrate (un-
        sweetened)*
    *all the ingredients of Orange Milk Sherbet (above)
        except orange juice*

Follow instructions for Orange Milk Sherbet. *Yield:* 8 ½-cup portions.

PINEAPPLE-ORANGE MILK SHERBET

½ 6-ounce can frozen pineapple juice concentrate (un-
     sweetened)
½ 6-ounce can frozen orange juice concentrate (unsweetened)
     all ingredients of Orange Milk Sherbet (facing page)
     except orange juice

Follow instructions for Orange Milk Sherbet. *Yield:* 8
½-cup portions.

PINEAPPLE-BANANA MILK SHERBET

1 6-ounce can frozen pineapple juice concentrate (un-
     sweetened)
1 cup mashed ripe bananas
     all ingredients of Orange Milk Sherbet (facing page)
     except orange juice
1 tablespoon ginger marmalade (optional)

Follow instructions for Orange Milk Sherbet. Add marmalade to mixture just before freezing. *Yield:* 10 ½-cup
portions.

FROZEN CUSTARD

1⅓ cups evaporated skim milk, chilled
2 teaspoons unflavored gelatin
4 tablespoons water
2 eggs, separated
6 tablespoons vegetable oil
4 tablespoons honey
½ cup chopped toasted almonds or crushed macaroons
1 teaspoon vanilla extract
2 tablespoons rum, brandy, or sherry (optional)
4 tablespoons sugar

Mix gelatin with water and heat to dissolve. Cool to room temperature. In small-bottomed chilled bowl beat egg yolks with fork while slowly adding oil drop by drop to make a smooth, thick mixture. Add honey, almonds (or macaroons), vanilla, liquor, and dissolved gelatin. Mix well. Beat egg whites stiff, gradually adding sugar while beating. Fold into egg yolks. Whip milk very stiff (see *Note* for Orange Milk Sherbet, page 138). Fold into egg mixture lightly but thoroughly. Pour at once into cold freezer tray. Freeze. *Yield:* 12 ½-cup portions.

BROILED PEACHES

4 large ripe peaches
1 pot boiling water
1 tablespoon brown sugar
1 tablespoon lemon juice
1 teaspoon margarine

Drop peaches one by one into boiling water, and remove after about 1 minute. Slip off skin. Cut in half, remove pits and discard them. Place in shallow pan, hollow side up. Sprinkle with sugar and lemon juice. Dot with margarine. Broil for 5 to 10 minutes or until tender and browned on top. Serve hot. *Yield:* Serves 4.

A BALKAN RECIPE

BALKAN EGGPLANT

1   *eggplant (1½ pounds)*
2   *tablespoons vegetable oil*
1   *medium onion, halved*
2   *tablespoons vinegar*
    salt to taste

Wash eggplant and place on pan in vertical position. Bake at 500° until soft to touch (10 to 15 minutes). Remove from oven. Holding eggplant with fork, peel quickly. Beat pulp with beater or electric mixer. With teaspoon, scrape juice from center of onion halves. Add to eggplant pulp. Add oil, vinegar, and salt. Mix well. Chill before serving. *Yield:* Serves 4.

BRITISH RECIPES

LONDON BROIL

2½   *pounds London broil (tender flank steak or rump of beef)*
 2   *tablespoons Worcestershire sauce*

Rub meat on both sides with sauce. Let stand 1 to 2 hours. Broil in preheated broiler to desired doneness. Slice thin. *Yield:* Serves 8.

FRUIT AND NUT CAKE

 1   *cup chopped walnuts*
 1   *cup chopped dates*
 1   *cup raisins*
 1   *teaspoon baking soda*
 1   *cup boiling water*
 ½   *cup sugar*
 ½   *cup oil*
1½   *cups sifted flour*
 2   *eggs*
 1   *teaspoon vanilla*
 ½   *teaspoon grated lemon rind*

Combine walnuts, dates, raisins, and baking soda. Add boiling water. Set aside. In mixing bowl, combine sugar and oil. Add flour, then eggs one at a time, blending well. Add vanilla and lemon rind. Stir in fruit and nut mixture. Turn into greased loaf pan. Bake in 350° oven until cake tests done (about 1½ hours). *Yield:* 1 cake.

CHINESE RECIPES

SWEET AND PUNGENT SAUCE

2	tablespoons vegetable oil
1	medium green pepper, cut into strips
1	carrot, cut into ¼-inch rounds
1½	teaspoons salt
3	tablespoons tomato ketchup
¼	cup sugar
¼	cup cider vinegar
½	cup water
1	cup drained pineapple chunks (optional)
1	tablespoon cornstarch, dissolved in
3	tablespoons water

Heat oil in skillet. Add green pepper and carrot. Sauté for 2 minutes. Add salt and mix well. Remove the vegetables and set aside. Using the same pan, add tomato ketchup and stir for 1 minute. Add sugar, vinegar, water, and pineapple chunks. Bring mixture to boil. Add the cooked vegetables and mix well. Add the cornstarch mixture and stir until transparent. *Serving suggestion:* Lends that Oriental something to broiled, panfried, or boiled fish, liver, and chicken. *Yield:* Serves 4.

STEAMED FISH

1   *pound fish (cod, striped bass, red snapper, or other*
      fillet or fish steak)
      salt
2   *stalks scallions, cut into 1-inch lengths*
½   *teaspoon ginger powder or fresh chopped ginger*

Sprinkle salt on each side of fish. Let stand 20 minutes. Rinse the fish in cold water. Pat dry with paper towel. Place half of scallions on heat-resistant plate. Add fish. Place remaining scallions and ginger on top of fish. Select a pot large enough to hold plate with fish. Add about 1½ inches of water to pot. Place a custard cup in center of pot. Bring water to boil. Set plate with fish on top of custard cup. Cover at once. Cook for 3 to 5 minutes. Turn heat off. Let stand covered for 5 minutes. Serve hot as is or with Sweet and Pungent Sauce (preceding recipe). *Yield:* Serves 4.

CHINESE BRAISED CHICKEN

1   *frying chicken, cut into serving-size pieces*
1   *clove garlic, crushed*
2   *tablespoons vegetable oil*
2   *tablespoons sherry*
2   *tablespoons soy sauce*
½   *pound whole mushroom caps*

Brown chicken and garlic lightly in oil. Add sherry and sauce, and cook for 3 minutes. Add mushroom caps.

Cover and simmer until tender (about 20 to 30 minutes). *Yield:* Serves 4.

FRENCH RECIPES

CRUDITÉS (Crisp, Colorful Raw Vegetables)

Raw vegetables cut into strips, slices or fancy shapes. Choose among carrots, celery, cucumbers, zucchini, white or yellow turnips, fennel, radishes, cauliflower, and broccoli flowerets.

Serving suggestion: These go well with dips (pages 130 to 131).

BÉCHAMEL-TYPE SAUCE (White Sauce)

2   *tablespoons vegetable oil*
2   *tablespoons flour*
1   *cup liquid low-fat milk*
    salt and pepper to taste

Heat oil. Add flour, cooking while stirring. Keep heat low so that flour mixture remains light in color. Do not brown. Stir in milk slowly. Bring to boil and cook for 2 to 3 minutes. Season with salt and pepper. *Note:* Broth, or vegetable or fish stock, may be used for all or part of the milk, depending on kind of food the sauce is to accompany. *Variations:* Vary the flavor by adding any one of the following: celery salt, onion juice, grated nutmeg, Worcestershire sauce, chopped chives, dill, or parsley. *Serving suggestion:* Adds richness to vegetables (broccoli, asparagus, cauliflower, and carrots), fish, and poultry. *Yield:* About 1 cup.

MAYONNAISE

1   *egg yolk*
1   *teaspoon prepared mustard*
½   *teaspoon salt*
    pinch pepper
½   *teaspoon sugar*
    pinch cayenne pepper
1   *cup vegetable oil*
    juice of ½ lemon

Chill well egg yolk, bowl, and wire whisk. Place bowl on wet paper towel to prevent spinning. Combine first 6 ingredients. Mix well with wire whisk. At first, add oil drop by drop to mixture, beating continuously. As mixture thickens, add oil in slow, steady stream, continuing to beat. Mix in lemon juice. Store in refrigerator in covered jar. *Serving suggestions:* Use in potato or macaroni salad, over cooked vegetables, such as broccoli, asparagus, and cauliflower, and over poached fresh salmon, halibut, scallops, and other fish and seafood (hot or cold). Also use in salads made with cooked chicken, veal or shrimp, canned tuna or salmon. *Yield:* About 1 cup.

FRENCH DRESSING

> 1   cup vegetable oil
> 1/4 cup apple cider vinegar
> 1   teaspoon sugar
> 1   teaspoon salt

Add all ingredients to bottle or jar. Cover tightly and shake well. Chill several hours. Shake thoroughly before serving. *Variations:* Substitute lemon juice for all or part of the vinegar. Add any or all of the following: 1/2 teaspoon paprika, 1/2 teaspoon dry mustard, 1 clove garlic (remove before dressing is stored). *Serving suggestions:* Use with raw salad greens, cooked string beans, asparagus, and broccoli. Also good as a marinade or basting liquid for meat and fish. *Yield:* 1 1/4 cups.

HERB DRESSING

> 1   cup French Dressing (*preceding recipe*)
> 1   teaspoon dried herbs of your choice, or
> 1   tablespoon fresh or dried herbs, including tarragon, chervil, chives, dill, sweet basil and oregano

Mix dressing and herbs. *Serving suggestions:* Use on sliced tomatoes, or tossed with raw salad greens. *Yield:* 1 cup.

RED OIL DRESSING

1   cup French Dressing (*preceding page*)
²/₃ cup ketchup
1   clove garlic, crushed

Mix all ingredients. *Serving suggestion:* Goes with tossed green salad. *Yield:* 1²/₃ cups.

FRENCH ONION SOUP

2   large onions, sliced thin
3   tablespoons vegetable oil
4   cups fat-free stock or broth
    salt and pepper
2   tablespoons grated Parmesan cheese

Sauté onions in heated oil until golden. Add stock and simmer ½ hour. Season with salt and pepper. Sprinkle with cheese before serving. *Yield:* Serves 4.

POACHED FISH

1½ pounds cod, halibut, salmon, whitefish, pike fillets
1½ teaspoons salt
2   cups water
1   medium onion
4   peppercorns
1   bay leaf
1   tablespoon lemon juice
1   tablespoon vinegar

Cut fish into serving pieces. Rub on salt lightly. Place fish in saucepan. Add water, onion, and seasonings. Bring to boil. Cover and simmer (do not boil) for about 15 minutes. *Serving suggestions:* Magnificent as is or with a sauce made from mayonnaise mixed with grated horseradish or capers to taste. Excellent, too, with tartar sauce. Recipe for mayonnaise is on page 146; tartar sauce recipe is on page 132. *Yield:* Serves 4.

SALMON STEAK BAKED IN WINE

 1 *pound fresh salmon slices, ½-inch thick*
    salt and pepper
½ *cup dry white wine or dry sherry*
    juice of ½ lemon
 1 *clove garlic, peeled and sliced (optional)*
 2 *tablespoons vegetable oil*

Preheat oven to 400°. Sprinkle salmon slices on all sides with salt and pepper. Place in baking pan. Combine remaining ingredients and pour over fish. Bake about 15 to 20 minutes, or when fish flakes easily when tested with a fork. Serve hot or cold. *Note:* Use same recipe with your favorite fish steaks as well as for whole fish, such as whitefish or striped bass. Adjust cooking time to weight and thickness of fish. *Yield:* Serves 3.

FRESH STRAWBERRIES WITH WINE

1   *quart fresh strawberries*
1/2 *cup Marsala or sauterne*
2   *tablespoons sugar*

Wash, hull, and chill strawberries. Chill wine and pour over berries. Just before serving, sprinkle with sugar. *Yield:* Serves 6.

ORANGES WITH KIRSCH OR PLUM BRANDY

4   *eating oranges*
2   *teaspoons sugar*
2   *teaspoons kirsch or plum brandy*

Peel and slice oranges. Remove seeds. In a bowl, arrange a layer of orange slices. Sprinkle with kirsch or brandy. Build additional layers and repeat until all slices have been sprinkled. *Yield:* Serves 4.

A HAWAIIAN RECIPE

SHRIMP HAWAIIAN STYLE

1   *pound raw shrimp*
3   *sliced scallions or 1 medium onion*
2   *tablespoons vegetable oil*
2   *tablespoons soy sauce*
1   *teaspoon salt*
¼   *teaspoon Tabasco sauce*
1   *cup fresh or bottled clam juice*
1   *teaspoon cornstarch*
1   *tablespoon water*

Shell and devein shrimp. Sauté scallions or onion in oil for 2 minutes. Add soy sauce, salt, Tabasco sauce, and clam juice. Cook over low heat for about 10 minutes. Mix cornstarch and water. Stir into hot mixture. Cook until thickened (about 1 minute). Add shrimp. Cover and simmer for about 8 minutes. *Serving suggestion:* Rice goes well with this dish. *Yield:* Serves 4.

HUNGARIAN RECIPES

CHICKEN PAPRIKA

2	medium onions, sliced
3	tablespoons vegetable oil
2-3	tablespoons paprika
1	frying chicken, cut into serving-size pieces
	salt and pepper
1	tablespoon flour
½	cup chicken broth or water
1	teaspoon lemon juice, or
1	tablespoon white wine

Preheat oven to 325°. Sauté onions in oil until golden. Add paprika and mix. Add chicken pieces, tossing them until well coated with onion. Sprinkle with salt and pepper. Cover and bake in pan for about 45 minutes. Remove chicken. Keep warm. Mix flour with chicken broth or water, and add pan juices. Add lemon juice or wine. Cook for 2 to 3 minutes. Pour over chicken. *Serving suggestion:* Delicious with rice or noodles. *Yield:* Serves 4.

VEAL GOULASH

1   *pound boneless veal*
3   *tablespoons flour*
1/2 *teaspoon salt*
    dash pepper
1   *tablespoon oil*
3/4 *cup thinly sliced onions*
1   *teaspoon paprika*
4   *ounces tomato sauce (page 133)*

Trim all visible fat from meat and discard. Cut veal into 1-inch cubes. Dip into mixture of flour, salt, and pepper. Heat oil in a Dutch oven. Sauté onions for about 10 minutes. Sprinkle with paprika. Add meat and brown well on both sides. Add tomato sauce. Cover and cook over low heat for 1 hour or until tender. *Yield:* Serves 4.

BAKED GINGER PEARS

4   *ripe pears*
1/2 *cup sugar (white or brown)*
1   *tablespoon lemon juice*
1/4 *cup white or red wine*
1   *1-inch slice ginger, or*
1/2 *teaspoon ground ginger*

Peel pears, cut in half, and core. Place in baking dish. Sprinkle with sugar and lemon juice. Add enough wine to barely cover bottom of dish. Add ginger. Cover and bake at 350° for 30 minutes or until tender. Serve hot or cold. *Yield:* Serves 4.

INDIAN RECIPES

CURRY SAUCE

¼	cup chopped onion
4	tablespoons vegetable oil
½	to 1 teaspoon curry powder
1	medium tart apple, peeled and chopped
1½	tablespoons flour
1	cup broth (chicken, beef, shrimp, or vegetable)
1	cup low-fat liquid milk
1	tablespoon lemon juice
	salt to taste

Sauté onion in oil until tender. Add curry powder and apple, and continue cooking over low heat for 10 minutes. Stir in flour and blend until smooth. Slowly add broth, then milk. Bring to boil. Cook for 5 minutes. Add lemon juice and salt to taste. *Serving suggestion:* Makes an exotic dish with fish or leftover veal or chicken. Curried dishes go best with bland rice. *Yield:* 1½ cups.

CURRIED SCALLOPS

3 tablespoons oil
½ clove garlic, crushed (optional)
1 small onion, chopped
1 pound scallops
1 teaspoon salt
2 teaspoons curry powder
3 tablespoons dry white wine
  chopped parsley

Heat oil in skillet. Sauté garlic and onion until golden. Add scallops and salt. Sauté for 2 minutes. Add curry and wine. Bring mixture to boil. Turn heat off. Sprinkle with chopped parsley. *Serving suggestion:* Rice makes this an authentic Indian dish. *Yield:* Serves 4.

ITALIAN RECIPES

ITALIAN MUSHROOMS OR ARTICHOKE HEARTS

1 can mushroom caps, or
1 can artichoke hearts
  Italian dressing (low-calorie commercial)

Marinate either vegetable in dressing for 2 to 3 minutes. Serve with party picks. *Yield:* Serves 8.

BROCCOLI AND BRUSSELS SPROUTS ITALIAN STYLE

1   *pound mixed broccoli and Brussels sprouts*
2   *tablespoons vegetable oil*
1   *clove garlic, crushed*
1/2   *teaspoon salt*
1/2   *cup broth (or use bouillon cube dissolved in water)*

Peel broccoli stems and cut diagonally into 1-inch sections. Slice each broccoli floweret into 2 or 3 pieces. Cut Brussels sprouts into halves or quarters. Heat oil in skillet or pan. Brown garlic in oil. Add vegetables and salt. Sauté for 3 minutes. Add broth. Cover and simmer until just crisp and tender (about 5 to 10 minutes). *Yield:* Serves 4.

SHRIMP SCAMPI STYLE

1   *pound raw large shrimp*

FOR THE MARINADE:

1   *clove garlic, crushed*
1   *teaspoon salt*
1/2   *teaspoon dry mustard*
1/4   *teaspoon pepper*
2   *tablespoons chopped parsley*
3   *tablespoons lemon juice*
1/4   *cup oil*

Shell and devein shrimp. Combine remaining ingredients. Pour over shrimp and let stand for 1 to 2 hours. Broil marinated shrimp about 4 inches from heat for about 4 minutes. *Serving suggestion:* Rice makes a proper Italian accompaniment. *Yield:* Serves 4.

CHICKEN MILANESE

1	*whole chicken breast*
1	*tablespoon flour*
1	*egg white, or*
1/2	*egg*
	salt, pepper, or ginger
3	*tablespoons fine bread crumbs*
1	*tablespoon grated Parmesan cheese*
2	*tablespoons oil*

Bone chicken breast and remove skin. Pound to flattten slightly. Dust with flour. Mix egg white or egg with salt, pepper, or ginger. Dip chicken breast into seasoned egg. Coat with crumbs mixed with cheese. Let stand 5 to 10 minutes. Heat oil. Brown chicken for about 5 minutes on each side. *Yield:* Serves 2.

VEAL AND PEPPERS

3   *medium green peppers, and*
1   *medium red pepper, seeded and cut into 1-inch strips*
4   *tablespoons vegetable oil*
1   *pound boneless veal (rump, shoulder, or leg), cut into 1½-inch pieces*
¼   *pound mushrooms, sliced*
1   *cup canned tomatoes, drained and slightly broken up with fork, or*
1   *cup tomato purée*
    black pepper

Sauté peppers in 2 tablespoons oil until brown or black spots develop (flavor is enhanced when this occurs). Remove from pan. In the same pan, brown veal cubes in residual oil. Add mushrooms and cook for about 10 minutes. Place veal mixture in baking dish. Add tomatoes, peppers, and black pepper to taste. Cover and bake in 325° oven for about 1 hour. *Yield:* Serves 4.

LIVER AND ONIONS VENETIAN STYLE

1   *pound beef liver*
4   *medium onions*
½   *teaspoon salt*
2   *tablespoons vegetable oil*
½   *cup white wine (optional)*

Cut liver into 1-inch cubes, discarding skin and veins. Cut onions into small pieces. Add salt and sauté in oil until golden. Add liver to onions. Cook and stir for about 3 minutes. Add wine just before serving. *Yield:* Serves 4

ITALIAN SEASONED CRUMBS

    1   cup bread crumbs
    1   teaspoon salt
    ¼   teaspoon pepper
    ¼   teaspoon oregano
    2   tablespoons grated Parmesan cheese

Mix all ingredients well. *Serving suggestion:* Adds that fine Italian taste to chicken, fish, and vegetables when used as a topping. *Yield:* 1 cup.

JAPANESE RECIPES

SOY SAUCE SAMURAI

- 1 *tablespoon vegetable oil*
- 2 *large scallions, cut into 1-inch lengths*
- 1 *teaspoon shredded ginger (optional)*
- 2 *teaspoons soy sauce*
- 1 *tablespoon water*

Heat oil. Add scallions and ginger. Cook until brown. Add soy sauce and water. Bring mixture to boil. Mix well. Remove from heat. *Serving suggestion:* Pour over steamed fish. *Yield:* Serves 4.

JAPANESE BARBECUED CHICKEN

- 1 *frying chicken, cut into quarters*

FOR THE MARINADE:

- 1/2 *teaspoon rosemary or poultry seasoning*
- 2 *tablespoons white wine or lemon juice*
- 1/2 *cup soy sauce*
- 1/4 *cup tomato ketchup*
- 2 *tablespoons oil*

Combine marinade ingredients. Marinate chicken 1 to 3 hours. Barbecue over charcoal or broil in oven. *Note:* Leftover marinade can be stored in refrigerator and reused within a short time. *Yield:* Serves 4.

JEWISH RECIPES

CHOPPED LIVER

$^1/_2$ pound liver (chicken, beef, or calves')
 2 tablespoons finely chopped onions
 2 tablespoons vegetable oil
 2 hard-cooked eggs, finely mashed
     salt and pepper
     any one or any combination of the following spices:
         cinnamon (pinch), allspice, marjoram, poultry sea-
         soning (optional)

Remove any attached fat from liver. Sauté onions in oil until well-browned. Add liver and cook gently until just done. Thoroughly chop or mash liver-and-onion mixture. Combine with eggs. Add seasonings. Mash well with fork. If additional moisture is needed, add a small amount of oil. *Serving suggestions:* Serve cold as a spread or dip, or on lettuce as an appetizer. *Yield:* Serves 8 as spread or dip; 4 as appetizer.

LOW-FAT "SOUR CREAM"

1/3   cup low-fat liquid milk or buttermilk
1   teaspoon lemon juice
1/4   teaspoon salt
1   8-ounce container cottage cheese

Place all ingredients in blender. Blend until completely
smooth. Refrigerate. *Variation:* Mix with your favorite
blend of herbs and spices. *Serving suggestions:* Use for
dips or, with chives or onion, on potatoes. Pour over
fruit. *Yield:* 1¼ cups.

A MEXICAN RECIPE

MEXICAN-STYLE BEANS

1   tablespoon oil
1   slice green pepper, chopped
1   slice onion, chopped
1   cup tomatoes, strained
1/2   teaspoon salt
1   clove garlic, minced (optional)
2/3   cup cooked dry kidney or lima beans
      parsley, chopped

Heat oil. Add chopped vegetables. Cook about 3 minutes.
Add tomatoes, salt, and a little garlic. When mixture
boils, add beans. Simmer 15 to 30 minutes. Add chopped
parsley before serving. *Yield:* Serves 2.

NEAR EASTERN RECIPES

NEAR EASTERN ROASTED GREEN PEPPER SALAD

4   *medium peppers*
4   *tablespoons vegetable oil*
4   *teaspoons vinegar*
     salt and pepper to taste
1   *clove garlic (optional)*

Preheat broiler. Broil peppers under medium heat in aluminum broiler pan, turning frequently with tongs, until skin has blackened on all sides and peppers are just tender. Place in bowl, cover tightly, and let stand for 10 to 20 minutes. This step helps you loosen and remove skin. Peel off blackened skin gently. Cut peppers lengthwise. Carefully remove seeds. Arrange peppers in bowl. Cover with dressing: 4 tablespoons oil, 4 teaspoons of vinegar, and salt and pepper to taste. Add garlic, peeled and halved. Refrigerate. *Note:* Peppers are at the peak of flavor after standing 2 to 3 days. *Yield:* Serves 4.

CHICKEN LIVER KEBOBS

1 *pound chicken livers*
2 *medium tomatoes, cut into wedges*
1 *large green pepper, cut into wedges*
2 *medium onions, cut into wedges, or*
8 *small button onions*
1 *small can pineapple chunks*

FOR THE MARINADE:
3 *tablespoons vegetable oil*
1/2 *teaspoon salt*
1/2 *teaspoon pepper*
1/4 *cup chopped onions*
1 *tablespoon Worcestershire sauce*

Pat chicken livers dry with paper towel. Combine ingredients for marinade. Marinate livers for 3 hours. Skewer livers alternately with vegetables and pineapple chunks. Broil for 10 minutes. Baste with remaining marinade, turning skewers 2 or 3 times during broiling. *Yield:* Serves 4.

PUERTO RICAN RECIPES

MARINATED GARBANZOS (Chick Peas)

  1 *1-pound can garbanzos, drained*
 ½ *cup vegetable oil*
  3 *tablespoons vinegar*
 ½ *cup fresh chopped parsley*
 ¼ *cup chopped scallions*
     dash garlic salt
     salt and pepper

Combine all ingredients. Marinate for at least 2 hours. Serve in bowl with party picks. *Yield:* 3 cups.

SOFRITO

  6 *tablespoons vegetable oil*
  2 *ounces cooked lean ham, chopped*
  3 *small sweet peppers, chopped*
  1 *onion, chopped*
  1 *clove garlic, chopped*
  1 *8-ounce can tomato sauce*
  3 *cilantro leaves (carried in Spanish grocery stores; use parsley or coriander if unavailable), chopped*

Heat oil. Sauté chopped ham. Add remaining ingredients. Reduce heat and simmer for 5 minutes. *Yield:* 1 cup.

PUERTO RICAN BEANS

1 *pound dried beans or pigeon peas*
1/2 *pound chopped raw pumpkin*
1/2 *cup Sofrito (preceding recipe)*
    salt and pepper to taste

Wash beans. Soak for about 6 hours or overnight. Bring bean-water mixture to boil, adding more water if necessary. Reduce heat and simmer until tender (about 1 hour). Add pumpkin and Sofrito. Stir in salt and pepper. Continue simmering until mixture thickens. *Serving suggestion:* Makes a filling dish when served over rice. *Yield:* Serves 10.

RUSSIAN RECIPES

RUSSIAN DRESSING

1 *cup mayonnaise (page 146)*
1/4 *cup chili sauce*
1/2 *teaspoon Worcestershire sauce*

Blend thoroughly. *Serving suggestion:* Adds tang to greens and seafood salads. *Yield:* 1¼ cups.

BORSCHT (Beet Soup)

1   *bunch young beets with greens*
2   *quarts boiling water*
     salt to taste
2   *eggs*
     juice of 1 lemon
     sugar to taste

Wash beets and beet greens thoroughly. Boil beets in water until they can be peeled easily (about 15 minutes). Cut them fine or grate on coarse grater. Chop greens. Cover beets and greens with boiling water. Add salt. Simmer until beets are tender (about 15 minutes). Beat eggs in a large bowl. Pour a small amount of borscht into eggs, stirring constantly to prevent curdling. Slowly add remainder of borscht. Add lemon juice and sugar. *Serving suggestion:* Traditionally this dish is served hot or cold with sour cream (see recipe for Low-Fat "Sour Cream," page 162) and hot boiled potatoes. *Yield:* Serves 6.

LOW-FAT YOGURT

  1   *cup non-fat dry milk*
  3   *cups water*
  1/4 *cup plain yogurt*

Mix milk and water. Bring to boil slowly. Cool to lukewarm. Thin out yogurt by adding ½ cup lukewarm milk. Stir well until smooth. Add yogurt mixture to rest of milk. Blend thoroughly. Pour into serving cups. Cover with thick paper towel. Place additional paper toweling between cups to maintain an even, warm temperature. Leave undisturbed for 5 to 6 hours, free from drafts and jolts. Refrigerate after yogurt solidifies. Set aside a small portion to start a new batch. *Note:* Initial batch contains less fat than commercial low-fat yogurts. Each succeeding batch contains less and less fat. After the third or fourth batch, the yogurt is virtually fat-free. *Variations:* Add sweet fresh or stewed fruit, berries, and sweet spices such as allspice and cinnamon. *Yield:* About 3¼ cups.

VIENNESE RECIPES

SPICED BAKED PRUNES

2   tablespoons brown sugar
1   tablespoon cornstarch
3   cups unsweetened orange juice
1   box (about 12 ounces) dried prunes
1   piece lemon peel
1   1-inch cinnamon stick
5   whole cloves (optional)
5   whole allspice (optional)
1/4 cup claret, port, or sherry

Mix sugar with cornstarch. Add orange juice. Place prunes in casserole. Pour orange juice mixture over prunes. Add lemon peel and spices. Cover and bake at 350° for 35 to 45 minutes. Remove from oven and add wine. *Serving suggestions:* Serve hot or cold as a dessert, or as an accompaniment to poultry or pork. *Yield:* Serves 12.

ORANGE CHIFFON CAKE

1	cup sifted cake flour
1½	teaspoons baking powder
¼	teaspoon salt
½	cup sugar
⅓	cup vegetable oil
1	egg yolk
⅓	cup orange juice
1	teaspoon vanilla
2	tablespoons grated orange rind
3	egg whites
¼	teaspoon cream of tartar
¼	cup sugar

Sift flour, baking powder, and salt in large bowl. Make a hole in center of flour and add sugar, oil, egg yolk, orange juice, vanilla, and orange rind. Beat until smooth. In another bowl combine egg whites with cream of tartar and sugar and beat until soft peaks form. Pour egg-yolk mixture gradually over beaten egg whites, folding gently with rubber scraper until just blended. Pour mixture into ungreased round 10-inch cake pan. Bake in 350° oven until top of cake springs back when touched lightly (about 30 minutes). Turn pan upside down. Let cool. Loosen cake from pan. *Yield:* 1 cake.

MEAL PLANNING WITH STAY-SLIM RECIPES

The Bureau of Nutrition, New York City Department of Health, has established the following guidelines for planning weight-control meals for the rest of your life:

· Include plenty of vegetables and fruits. Preferred are dark-green leafy vegetables (salad greens) and yellow vegetables (carrots, pumpkins, sweet potatoes, and winter squash) for their high vitamin A and C content.

· Include bread and unsweetened cereals. They are low in fat and *non-fattening* when eaten in moderation.

· Include high-protein foods, such as fish, lean meat, poultry, low-fat cheese, and low-fat milk. Eggs, a high-protein food, are also high in cholesterol and should be limited to four a week.

· Replace table and cooking fats (butter, lard, and shortenings) with vegetable oils (corn, safflower, and so on), or with margarines containing a substantial amount of liquid oil.

And—

· *Treat yourself to a high-calorie dessert on special occasions, or have a candy bar or an ice cream soda once in a while.* It won't show on the scale provided you stick to the I Love New York Lifetime Stay-Slim Program at all other times. Amazing but true!

14

Common Sense About Exercise, Weight Loss, and Health

ON THE I LOVE NEW YORK DIET PROGRAM you don't have to exercise to look like a glamorous member of the jet set, but exercise is so beneficial in so many ways that the Bureau of Nutrition, New York City Department of Health, strongly recommends it.

But doesn't exercise increase the appetite, and end up putting weight on you?

No, answers Dr. Lawrence V. Oscat, Associate Professor of Physical Education at the University of Illinois. "Exercise does not increase appetite. Controlled studies with humans and animals refute this long-held myth."

As a matter of fact, adds Dr. Jeremiah Stamler, Chairman of the Department of Community Health and

Preventive Medicine, Northwestern University Medical School, "many people [who exercise] tend to eat *less*."

The type of exercise to which Drs. Oscat and Stamler refer is short term. Of course, if you're a lumberjack your appetite at the end of a workday is as big as a redwood. But exercising an hour or so a day, which is sufficient for most adults, is not an appetite stimulant. Nobody has ever gained weight from short-term exercise. Almost everybody loses weight from it.

EXERCISE SPEEDS WEIGHT LOSS, HELPS KEEP IT OFF WHILE YOU EAT MORE

Short-term exercise (from now on whenever exercise is mentioned, read short-term exercise) cannot slim you down rapidly, nor can it keep you slim permanently. It works only when accompanied by sound nutritional habits—the habits you learn on the I Love New York Diet Program.

When I (Bill) was reducing I walked briskly to my office each morning and back to my apartment each evening—a total distance of about five miles, which I covered in about an hour and a half. I used up about six calories each walking minute—a total of 540 calories a day and 3,240 calories in a six-day week. To lose a pound of fat, anybody must expend about 3,500 calories. I lost almost an extra pound every week.

Since I've been at my ideal weight, I've continued to

walk briskly to and from work. But I haven't continued to lose that extra pound a week. I just make up the calories I expend walking by eating more. My weight stays rocksteady while I enjoy the luxury of extra portions of my favorite foods.

THE BEST TYPE OF EXERCISE

Brisk walking promotes circulatory fitness. Other exercises of this type include jogging, running, swimming, bicycling, bowling, rope skipping, tennis, and dancing. These exercises, according to physical fitness expert Ronald M. Deutsch, "are the ones which burn most calories ... with the least fatigue."

You can also get this medically approved type of exercise from working hard around the house or in the garden, or from climbing stairs. But you're not likely to get it at your job. "The muscular effort required by most jobs in this country is negligible," asserts Dr. Joseph T. Doyle of the Albany (N.Y.) Medical College. Nor can you get it from isometric (stationary) exercises and weight lifting. These exercises develop some muscles, but do not provide the general body motion that improves blood circulation.

The best kind of exercise for you is one that gets your whole body moving. Pick the specific one that's most fun to do. If it's golf, say no to the golf cart.

HOW MUCH EXERCISE YOU NEED TO LOSE ONE POUND A WEEK

The figures in the following chart are approximations for a person weighing about 150 pounds. The heavier you are, the less exercise time you need to drop a pound; the lighter you are, the more exercise time you need. As a rule of thumb, if you're over 150 pounds, decrease the exercise times in the chart by 10 percent; if you're under 150 pounds, increase them by 10 percent.

HOURS OF EXERCISE TIME REQUIRED TO LOSE ONE POUND

Dancing (disco)	3½
Running	3½
Skating (ice or roller)	5
Jogging	6
Bicycling (fast)	6
Walking	10
Dancing (ballroom)	10
Swimming	4½
Skiing	5
Tennis	6
Table tennis	7

Bowling	10
Golf (no cart)	10
Gardening	10
Housework	10
Climbing stairs	10

EXERCISE AWAY ONE POUND A WEEK AND ENJOY THESE SPECIAL EATING TREATS

To hold your weight steady when you exercise away a pound a week, you can eat up to 3,500 calories more per week of anything you like. Here's what one weekly 3,500-calorie "binge-while-you-stay-slim" menu looks like:

- A large scoop of ice cream, and
- A milk shake or malted milk, and
- An order of pancakes with syrup, and
- A slice of apple pie with Cheddar cheese, and
- A glazed doughnut, and
- A hamburger on a bun with trimmings, and
- A pork chop, and
- A sirloin steak, and
- An order of corn flakes with whole milk, and
- A regular soft drink, and
- An extra bottle of beer, and—as a tribute to the I Love New York Diet and Exercise Program, which makes this no-weight-gain binging possible—
- A Big Apple

THE HEALTH-PROMOTING QUALITIES OF EXERCISE

Medical opinion holds that exercise on a daily basis—

- Relieves feelings of stress and anxiety, and increases feelings of well-being and confidence
- Improves stamina
- Helps keep hypertension (high blood pressure) and diabetes under control
- Decreases heartbeat rate over a twenty-four hour period, thus putting less strain on the heart
- Tones up muscles, including the heart muscle
- Relieves fatigue and makes it easier to sleep
- Helps replace flabby fat tissue with firm muscle tissue
- Fights stiffness in the joints, arthritic symptoms, and other signs of aging
- Helps prevent general aches and pains
- Improves digestion and disposition
- And it may increase the blood level of high-density lipoproteins, which combat heart attack

DOS AND DON'TS FOR THE BEGINNING EXERCISER

· *Do* get your doctor's advice before embarking on an exercise program. Dr. Lenore R. Zohman, Associate Professor of Rehabilitative Medicine at the Albert Einstein College of Medicine and a leading expert on exercise therapy, advises that "a sedentary prospective exerciser should have a checkup by his physician, including an examination of the cardiovascular system, blood pressure, muscles and joints. His blood should be analyzed for cholesterol and triglycerides, and a resting electrocardiogram should be evaluated. Most importantly, the examination...should include an exercise stress test." *Don't* think you can exercise like a pro because *you* think you're in shape. Let your doctor decide.

· *Do* warm up with five minutes or so of light calisthenics before you plunge into any exercise, including housework. *Don't* exercise cold. It could lead to heart strain and injuries to muscles and bones.

· *Do* start your program with light exercise, such as walking or mild jogging. *Don't* rush into competitive sports like tennis. The desire to win can push you into overtaxing your body.

· *Do* increase the intensity and duration of your exercise gradually. *Don't* think you can walk long distances briskly or jog for miles energetically the first day.

· *Do* exercise at the time of day when you feel up.

Don't exercise when you're tired. Never exercise when you feel ill.

· *Do* exercise on an empty stomach. *Don't* drink alcohol before or after exercising.

· *Do* exercise outdoors only in clement weather. *Don't* exercise outdoors on hot, humid days or when the air quality is poor.

· *Do* start jogging on a soft surface (grass or cinder track). *Don't* start jogging on streets and highways until you've broken in your leg muscles on softer surfaces.

· *Do* continue exercising as long as it makes you feel good. *Don't* continue to exercise when you start feeling fatigue, perspire too heavily, can't catch your breath, get a pain in your chest, or feel distressed in any way.

· *Do* taper off for at least five minutes toward the end of your exercise period. *Don't* quit cold turkey. You could feel faint or dizzy.

15

The Hassle-Free Way To Better Health for the Rest of Your Life

THE I LOVE NEW YORK DIET, unlike most fad diets, is health promoting.

The Prudent Diet, on which the I Love New York Diet is based in large part, was designed by Dr. Jolliffe, the founder of the Bureau of Nutrition, New York City Department of Health, to combat heart attack and other nutrition-related diseases, not just obesity.

It is based on the inclusion of adequate fiber, and on the controlled use of fat, saturated fat, cholesterol, sugar, and salt—nutrients which have been indicated as potentially harmful when ingested in excessive quantities. The indictment comes from the U.S. Department of Agriculture and the U.S. Department of Health, Education, and Welfare, as well as from the Bureau of Nutrition.

This diet alone cannot guarantee perfect health. Too

many other factors—including infection, mental attitude, heredity, personality, environmental pollution, and stress—affect our bodies and our minds. But this diet, according to the Bureau of Nutrition's medical experts, can ward off nutrition-related diseases, keep you healthy, and even improve your health.

THIS DIET CUTS RATE OF HEART ATTACK, OTHER DISEASES, IN REAL-LIFE TEST

Most information about diets comes from patients observed under clinical conditions. The results obtained cannot always be duplicated in real life. But in a pioneering test conducted by the Bureau of Nutrition, 400 men on the Prudent Diet were permitted to live in their own homes and carry out their normal work and leisure activities. In this real-life test, the incidence of heart attack was cut by 500 percent! "A method that could effectively combat the coronary epidemic had been scientifically demonstrated," concluded the eminent nutritionist Dr. Arthur Blumenfeld.

Dr. Blumenfeld added that the diet had been adopted by numerous diabetes clinics and that "other metabolic ailments are normalized by [it]." These ailments include artery blockage of all types, arteriosclerosis (a thickening of the artery walls resulting in a diminished blood supply), gout, gallstones, cataracts (the clouding of the lens of the eye), *arcus senilis* (cholesterol deposits in the outer rim of the iris of the eye), and yellow atrophy of the liver. They also include hypertension (high blood pressure), hyperglycemia (high blood sugar), hypoglycemia (low blood sugar), diverticulosis (a disorder of the large bowel affecting many older people), constipation (a condition induced by many fad diets), and exotic lipid (fat and cholesterol) diseases, the symptoms of which are bumps in the skin, elbows, tendons, and other parts of the body.

"But have any *harmful* side effects been noticed?" Dr. Blumenfeld asks. He replies: "Doctors, researchers, statisticians, technicians, and nurses from New York to Los Angeles...answer 'No.' There is no illness (known or hidden) which can be aggravated by the diet."

Dr. Blumenfeld also reminds us that "the diet is medically recognized as the best type of reducing diet."

On the I Love New York Lifetime Stay-Slim Program, you have a choice of all the foods available to Americans—the widest choice ever known. Choose prudently, and your chance of staying slim, vigorous, and healthy will be improved significantly. You already know what foods are good for you—they're the ones you've been eating on the I Love New York reducing and maintenance diets.

FOODS THE BUREAU OF NUTRITION RECOMMENDS YOU EAT SPARINGLY FOR THE SAKE OF YOUR HEALTH

· *High-fat foods*. You can see most of the fat on meat, poultry, and fish, and can trim it away. But there are foods containing hidden fat, and there's nothing you can do about lowering *their* fat content. These foods include:

Avocados
Muffins
Biscuits
Danish pastry
Cookies
Doughnuts
Cakes and pies
Whole milk
Cream (sweet and sour)
Milk puddings
Butter
Butter substitutes
Cream cheese and other high-fat cheeses
Non-dairy cream substitutes

· *Saturated-fat foods.* There are three kinds of fats: saturated, polyunsaturated, and monosaturated. Saturated fats have been linked to nutrition-related diseases. Polyunsaturated fats are known to help ward off these diseases. Monosaturated fats are neutral. Saturated fats, which come mainly from animal sources, are solid at room temperature. Polyunsaturated fats, which are present in large quantities in fish and vegetable oils, are liquid at room temperature.

Watch out for these saturated-fat foods:

Meat—beef, lamb, pork, veal, and their products,
    such as cold cuts and sausages
Eggs
Whole milk
Whole-milk cheese
Cream (sweet and sour)
Ice cream
Butter
Some margarines (read the labels)
Lard
Hydrogenated shortenings
Chocolate
Coconut
Coconut oil
Palm oil
Products made from the items listed, such as cakes,
    pastry, cookies, gravies, sauces, and many commer-
    cial snack foods

· *High-cholesterol foods.* Cholesterol is a fatlike substance
essential to the well-being of every cell in the body. But
high levels of cholesterol in the blood may lead to heart
attack and other nutrition-related diseases. There is a
controversy about *how much* ingested cholesterol is dangerous, but most medical authorities agree that we
should limit our intake of such high-cholesterol foods
as:

Lard
Eggs

Cream (sweet or sour)
Liver
Butter (regular or whipped)
Sweetbreads
Pork spareribs
Duck
Kidneys
Brains

The following foods contain cholesterol in lesser amounts than those in the preceding list and may be eaten more frequently:

Oysters
Salmon
Scallops
Clams
Tuna
Halibut
Swordfish
Pork (other than spareribs)
Beef
Lobster
Poultry
Lamb
Crab
Cheese
Shrimp
Sardines

· *High-sugar foods.* Sugar is regarded as the prime example of an empty-calorie food—one which supplies calories but no nutritive value. Excess sugar has been associated by some researchers with nutrition-related diseases. The major hazard from too much sugar, according to the U.S. Department of Agriculture, is tooth decay. The average American consumes about 130 pounds of sugar a year, almost all of it hidden in prepared foods. It's health wise to cut down on these foods. Here's a list:

Jams
Jellies
Candies
Cookies
Cakes
Pies
Canned goods (read the labels)
Breakfast cereals
Ketchup and other condiments
Flavored milks and yogurt
Ice cream
Frozen prepared foods

• *High-salt foods.* Most of the salt we consume, like most of the fat and sugar, comes hidden in cooked or prepared food. Sodium is one of the constituents of salt; and scientists measure the amount of salt in food by its sodium content. A high-sodium diet has in some cases been related to the onset of hypertension (high blood pressure), the "silent killer" which afflicts 17 percent of the population of the United States. You can lower your chances of becoming a victim of hypertension by curbing your use of the salt shaker in the dining room and the kitchen, and by eating the following foods high in hidden salt only now and then:

Chocolate milk drinks
Buttermilk (with salt added)
Milk substitutes
Instant cocoa
Fruit-flavored drinks
Commercial breads, rolls, and biscuits
Popovers
Pancakes
Waffles
Pretzels, breadsticks, and salted crackers
Breakfast cereals
Self-rising flour
Regular salted cheese
Regular salted butter and margarine
Commercial mayonnaise and salad dressings
Cream substitutes
Bacon and other cured or smoked meat, poultry, and
    fish
Preseasoned meats (sausages, luncheon meats, corned
    beef, pastrami, and other delicatessen foods)
Frozen fish
Brains, heart, kidneys, and other organ meats
Commercial soups, soup mixes, and bouillon cubes
Potato chips and instant potatoes
Minute rice
Frozen candied sweets
Frozen peas and lima beans
Pickles and pickled foods

Condiments and relishes
MSG-seasoned foods

The following vegetables are naturally high in sodium but can be enjoyed fairly often, except by people on a low-sodium diet:

Beets
Beet greens
Swiss chard
Celery
Spinach

THE I LOVE NEW YORK DIET IS AN IMPROVEMENT OVER THE AVERAGE AMERICAN DIET

On the 7-day Crash Program and the Eating Holiday— *Fats are cut* to about 30 percent of the total calories consumed—some 15 percent less than most Americans are accustomed to eating. Low fat means low weight and a decreased chance of contracting a nutrition-related disease.

Polyunsaturated fats are increased from about 20 percent of the total fat content of the average diet to approximately 60 percent. Polyunsaturated fats help ward off nutrition-related diseases.

Cholesterol is reduced to about 360 milligrams a day—

approximately half the average American's consumption. Low cholesterol reduces the chances of heart attack and other metabolic diseases.

Carbohydrates are slashed from about 50 percent of the average American diet to approximately 35 percent. Lowered carbohydrate intake hastens weight loss.

Fiber is boosted from the less than 5 grams a day which we usually eat to 15 grams or more. High fiber protects against certain maladies of the digestive tract, including constipation.

Sugar is decreased from 18 percent of the total calories of our normal diet to about 10 percent. Sugar is an empty-calorie food associated by some medical authorities with nutrition-related diseases.

Sodium is minimized. The average American consumes from 7,000 to 10,000 milligrams a day, as compared with only about 3,000 milligrams on this diet. Excess sodium intake can lead in some cases to hypertension (high blood pressure) and in many cases to water bloat.

The Lifetime Stay-Slim Program is designed to keep you at your ideal weight healthfully. To do that, the nutritional statistics are adjusted to include about 16 percent protein and about 54 percent carbohydrates. All other nutritional statistics remain the same as on the reducing parts of the diet.

16

No-Calorie, Almost No-Calorie, and High-Fiber Foods

ON THE I LOVE NEW YORK DIET, you don't count calories and you're not going to start now. But you should know which foods you can eat and drink with no, or almost no, danger of weight gain. Following are lists of delectables with zero calories, with 1 to 15 calories, and with 16 to 25 calories. Here also is a list of foods that fill you up fast without threatening your waistline—high-fiber foods. Browse through these lists (you'll even find a chocolate cookie) and add variety to your Lifetime Stay-Slim Program. Quantities are normal, restaurant-size portions except where noted.

NO-CALORIE FOODS

Coffee	Herb teas
Tea	Bouillon
Mineral water	Clear soups
Diet soda	Consommé
Seltzer	All herbs and spices

1- TO 15-CALORIE FOODS

Asparagus	Mustard greens
Bean sprouts	Parsley
Beet greens	Peppers (green and red)
Broccoli	Pickles
Cabbage	Pimentos
Cauliflower	Radishes
Celery	Rhubarb
Collard greens	Sauerkraut
Cucumbers	Spinach
Dandelion greens	Squash
Endives	String beans
Escarole	Swiss chard
Kale	Turnip greens
Lettuce	Watercress
Mushrooms	

16- to 25-CALORIE FOODS

(COMMERCIAL)

1 Bacon Thin
1 cheese-flavored cracker
1 Oysterette
1 Melba Round
1 Wheat Thin
1 pizza-flavored cracker
1 shredded wheat, spoon-size

2 tablespoons reconstituted lemon juice
2 tablespoons reconstituted lime juice

1 cube beef bouillon
1 cube chicken bouillon
1 cube vegetable bouillon
1 serving canned beef broth
1 package instant beef broth
1 package instant vegetable broth

½ cup canned Chinese vegetables

1 olive
1 cocktail onion
1 midget gherkin

1   arrowroot cookie
1   chocolate cookie (Sunshine wafer)
1   graham cracker

1   tablespoon aerosol-canned whipped cream
1   tablespoon aerosol-canned dairy whip
1   teaspoon half-and-half (non-dairy creamer)

1   teaspoon extracts and flavorings

1   piece chewing gun

1   piece cocktail gefilte fish (in jars)
1   cocktail meatball (canned)

FRUIT

Cantaloupe   Lemon juice
Cranberries   Lime
Currants   Lime juice
Gooseberries   Strawberries
Honeydew melon   Watermelon
Lemon

VEGETABLES

Bamboo shoots   Eggplant
Beets   Fennel
Brussels sprouts   Kohlrabi
Carrots   Leeks

Okra
Scallions
Tomatoes

Tomato juice
Turnips

HIGH-FIBER FOODS

Almonds
Apples
Apricots
Asparagus
Bamboo shoots
Bananas
Beans, dry or fresh
Bean sprouts
Berries
Bran
Bread, whole-wheat
Brussels sprouts
Buckwheat groats (kasha)
Buckwheat, whole grain
Cabbage
Carrots
Cauliflower

Chestnuts
Cranberries
Dates
Figs
Lentils
Nuts
Okra
Oranges
Parsnips
Peas
Pea pods
Peanuts
Peppers, red and green
Popcorn
Sesame seeds
Wheat germ

Afterword

The Prudent Diet, on which the I Love New York Diet is based in part, was developed in 1958 by Dr. Norman Jolliffe, director, the Bureau of Nutrition, New York City Department of Health. Prior to that time Dr. Jolliffe served as a member of the Food and Nutrition Board of the National Research Council, as a member of the Board of the National Vitamin Foundation, and as an Associate Professor at the School of Public Health, Columbia University (New York). He contributed more than 200 articles on nutrition to scientific journals, and coauthored *Chemical Nutrition,* then the standard textbook in its field.

The I Love New York Diet 7-Day Crash Diet is based on Dr. Jolliffe's 600-calorie-a-day diet (which, because of larger portions on our diet, actually works out to about 1,000 to 1,200 calories a day), and the I Love

New York Eating Holiday on his 1,800-calorie-a-day diet. Two 2,000-calorie-a-day diets form the basis for the I Love New York Lifetime Stay-Slim Program: Dr. Jolliffe's and the maintenance diet recommended by the Bureau of Nutrition in its recent publications (1972–1981). The behavioral dietetics incorporated into the overall I Love New York Diet Program are based on the suggestions of Dr. Jolliffe, the work of his disciples, and the findings of numerous behavioral psychologists.

Recommended Reading

Dietary Goals for the United States, second edition. The United States Senate Select Committee on Nutrition and Human Needs makes its recommendations for a healthier America. Request current price of Stock No. 052-070-04376-8 and order from Superintendent of Documents, U.S. Government Printing Office, Washington, D.C. 20402.

Healthy People. The Surgeon-General's Report on health promotion and disease prevention. Request current price of Stock No. 017-001-00416-2 and order from Superintendent of Documents, U.S. Government Printing Office, Washington, D.C. 20402.

Heart Attack: Are You a Candidate? (1964) by Dr. Arthur Blumenfeld. The first and still the best popular exposition of how the basic diet described in this book fights coronary disease and a host of nutrition-related maladies. Out of print, but you may still be able to get a copy in your library. Worth hunting for. Published by Paul S. Ericksson, Inc., 119 West 57th Street, New York, N.Y. 10019.

The Dieter's Gourmet Cookbook (1979), *Diet for Life* (1980), and *Francine Prince's New Gourmet Recipes for Dieters* (1981) by Francine Prince, a national leading authority on cooking for better health. These three books together contain over 500 miraculously delicious low-calorie recipes that are also low in fat and in saturated fat and cholesterol, with no sugar or salt. Strongly recommended for any dieter. Published by Cornerstone Library, division of Simon & Schuster, Inc., 1230 Avenue of the Americas, New York, N.Y. 10020.

Nutrition and Health is a six-times-a-year newsletter that keeps you abreast of recent developments. Write for the current price and order from Institute of Human Nutrition, Columbia University College of Physicians and Surgeons, 701 West 168th Street, New York, N.Y. 10032.

Eat Right to Stay Healthy (1979) by Dr. Denis Burkitt answers many of your questions about fiber. Published by Arco Publishing Co., Inc., 219 Park Avenue South, New York, N.Y. 10003.

Vitamins and You (1979) by Robert J. Benowicz is far and away the best popular book on the how, what, why, when, and where of vitamins. Invaluable to any dieter. Published by Grosset & Dunlap, Inc., 51 Madison Avenue, New York, N.Y. 10010.

Sodium in Food, Medicine, and Water by Richard Weickart. A must for sodium watchers. It's free from the publisher, Water Quality Association, 477 East Butterfield Road, Lombard, Ill. 60148.

How Drinking Can Be Good for You (1978) by Dr. Morris C. Chafetz. Just what it says. Published by Stein and Day Publishers, Scarborough House, Braircliff Manor, N.Y. 10510.

Permanent Weight Control (1976) by Dr. Michael J. Mahoney and Kathryn Mahoney. All you would want to know about conditioning techniques that keep your weight off by altering your behavior patterns. Published by W. W. Norton & Co., Inc., 500 Fifth Avenue, New York, N.Y. 10036.

Index of Stay-Slim Gourmet Recipes

Scoreboards and
Restaurant Order Forms

THE I LOVE NEW YORK DIET
7-DAY CRASH PROGRAM
SCOREBOARD

YOUR WEIGHT

☐

Present Weight

DAYS ON DIET		DAILY WEIGHT LOSS
1	☐	☐
2	☐	☐
3	☐	☐
4	☐	☐
5	☐	☐
6	☐	☐
7	☐	☐

NEW SLIMMED-DOWN WEIGHT _____

☐

**WEIGHT LOSS
IN JUST ONE
WEEK**

THE I LOVE NEW YORK DIET
7-DAY CRASH PROGRAM
SCOREBOARD

YOUR WEIGHT

☐

Present Weight

DAYS ON DIET		DAILY WEIGHT LOSS
1	☐	☐
2	☐	☐
3	☐	☐
4	☐	☐
5	☐	☐
6	☐	☐
7	☐	☐

NEW SLIMMED-DOWN WEIGHT _____

☐

**WEIGHT LOSS
IN JUST ONE
WEEK**

THE I LOVE NEW YORK DIET
7-DAY CRASH PROGRAM
SCOREBOARD

YOUR WEIGHT

[ ]

Present Weight

DAYS ON DIET   **DAILY WEIGHT LOSS**

1	[ ]	[ ]
2	[ ]	[ ]
3	[ ]	[ ]
4	[ ]	[ ]
5	[ ]	[ ]
6	[ ]	[ ]
7	[ ]	[ ]

NEW SLIMMED-DOWN WEIGHT _____

[ ]

**WEIGHT LOSS
IN JUST ONE
WEEK**

THE I LOVE NEW YORK DIET
7-DAY CRASH PROGRAM
SCOREBOARD

YOUR WEIGHT

Present Weight

DAYS ON DIET		DAILY WEIGHT LOSS
1		
2		
3		
4		
5		
6		
7		

NEW SLIMMED-DOWN WEIGHT _____

**WEIGHT LOSS
IN JUST ONE
WEEK**

THE I LOVE NEW YORK
EATING HOLIDAY SCOREBOARD

YOUR WEIGHT

Present Weight

DAYS ON DIET		DAILY WEIGHT LOSS
1		
2		
3		
4		
5		
6		
7		

NEW SLIMMED-DOWN WEIGHT _____

WEIGHT LOSS
IN JUST ONE
WEEK

THE I LOVE NEW YORK DIET
EATING HOLIDAY SCOREBOARD

YOUR WEIGHT

☐

Present Weight

DAYS ON DIET		DAILY WEIGHT LOSS
1	☐	☐
2	☐	☐
3	☐	☐
4	☐	☐
5	☐	☐
6	☐	☐
7	☐	☐

NEW SLIMMED-DOWN WEIGHT _____

☐

**WEIGHT LOSS
IN JUST ONE
WEEK**

THE I LOVE NEW YORK
EATING HOLIDAY SCOREBOARD

YOUR WEIGHT

Present Weight

DAYS ON DIET		DAILY WEIGHT LOSS
1		
2		
3		
4		
5		
6		
7		

NEW SLIMMED-DOWN WEIGHT _____

WEIGHT LOSS
IN JUST ONE
WEEK

THE I LOVE NEW YORK
EATING HOLIDAY SCOREBOARD

YOUR WEIGHT

Present Weight

DAYS ON DIET		DAILY WEIGHT LOSS
1		
2		
3		
4		
5		
6		
7		

NEW SLIMMED-DOWN WEIGHT _____

**WEIGHT LOSS
IN JUST ONE
WEEK**

THE I LOVE NEW YORK
7-DAY CRASH DIET
RESTAURANT ORDER FORMS

BREAKFAST MENUS

CLIP AND PRESENT TO WAITER

DAY 1: BREAKFAST   THE I LOVE NEW YORK
7-DAY CRASH DIET

Orange
Egg, boiled or poached
Piece Melba toast
Coffee or tea

DAY 2: BREAKFAST   THE I LOVE NEW YORK
7-DAY CRASH DIET

Grapefruit
Cottage cheese (or low-fat pot cheese)
Coffee or tea

DAY 3: BREAKFAST   THE I LOVE NEW YORK
7-DAY CRASH DIET

Orange
Puffed wheat (preferably with no salt added)
Low-fat milk
Coffee or tea

DAY 4: BREAKFAST

THE I LOVE NEW YORK
7-DAY CRASH DIET

Grapefruit
Shredded wheat
Low-fat milk
Coffee or tea

DAY 5: BREAKFAST

THE I LOVE NEW YORK
7-DAY CRASH DIET

Tangerine or orange
1/2 thin-slice bread
Low-fat milk
Coffee or tea

DAY 6: BREAKFAST

THE I LOVE NEW YORK
7-DAY CRASH DIET

Grapefruit
Egg, boiled or poached
Piece RyKrisp
Coffee or tea

DAY 7: BREAKFAST

THE I LOVE NEW YORK
7-DAY CRASH DIET

Orange
Shredded wheat
Low-fat milk
Coffee or tea

LUNCH MENUS

CLIP AND PRESENT TO WAITER

DAY 1: LUNCH   THE I LOVE NEW YORK
7-DAY CRASH DIET

Shrimp or seafood of your choice
Celery, lettuce, tomatoes, and carrot sticks
Coffee, tea, or diet soda

DAY 2: LUNCH   THE I LOVE NEW YORK
7-DAY CRASH DIET

Sliced roast beef
Lettuce, celery, and tomatoes
Coffee, tea, or diet soda

DAY 3: LUNCH   THE I LOVE NEW YORK
7-DAY CRASH DIET

Fresh fruit salad
Cottage cheese
Coffee, tea, or diet soda

DAY 4: LUNCH THE I LOVE NEW YORK
7-DAY CRASH DIET

*Canned fish, such as tuna (oil removed, or packed in water
or broth)*
Lettuce, cucumbers, celery, and radishes
Coffee, tea, or club soda with lemon or lime

DAY 5: LUNCH THE I LOVE NEW YORK
7-DAY CRASH DIET

Broiled hamburger
Green salad with sliced tomatoes
Coffee, tea, or diet soda

DAY 6: LUNCH THE I LOVE NEW YORK
7-DAY CRASH DIET

Chicken or turkey slices
Lettuce, celery, and tomatoes
Coffee, tea, or diet soda

DAY 7: LUNCH THE I LOVE NEW YORK
7-DAY CRASH DIET

Sliced hard-cooked eggs
Mixed green salad
Coffee, tea, or diet soda

DINNER MENUS

CLIP AND PRESENT TO WAITER

DAY 1: DINNER   THE I LOVE NEW YORK
7-DAY CRASH DIET

Fresh fruit cocktail
Sautéed chicken breasts
Cabbage, turnips, and zucchini (or Brussels sprouts)
Coffee, tea, or club soda with lemon or lime

DAY 2: DINNER   THE I LOVE NEW YORK
7-DAY CRASH DIET

Tomato juice or V-8 (preferably with no salt added)
Broiled liver
Spinach, cauliflower, celery, and green pepper
Coffee, tea, or club soda with lemon or lime

DAY 3: DINNER   THE I LOVE NEW YORK
7-DAY CRASH DIET

Clams
Flounder, haddock, or fish of your choice
Celery, radishes, carrots, and zucchini (or cabbage)
Coffee, tea, or club soda with lemon or lime

DAY 4: DINNER THE I LOVE NEW YORK
7-DAY CRASH DIET

Roast veal
Mixed green salad
Strawberries or other berries in season
Coffee, tea, or club soda with lemon or lime

DAY 5: DINNER THE I LOVE NEW YORK
7-DAY CRASH DIET

Broiled chicken
Asparagus, spinach, and cauliflower
Fresh fruit salad
Coffee, tea, or club soda with lemon or lime

DAY 6: DINNER THE I LOVE NEW YORK
7-DAY CRASH DIET

Steak or London broil
Broccoli, string beans, and green peppers
Strawberries
Coffee, tea, or club soda with lemon or lime

DAY 7: DINNER THE I LOVE NEW YORK
7-DAY CRASH DIET

Crabmeat or seafood of your choice
Spinach, broccoli, and carrots
Grapefruit
Coffee, tea, or club soda with lemon or lime

THE I LOVE NEW YORK EATING HOLIDAY RESTAURANT ORDER FORMS

BREAKFAST MENUS

CLIP AND PRESENT TO WAITER

DAY 1: BREAKFAST   THE I LOVE NEW YORK
EATING HOLIDAY

Pineapple juice
Slice whole-wheat toast with margarine (diet margarine preferred)
Cream of wheat
Low-fat milk
Raisins
Coffee or tea

DAY 2: BREAKFAST   THE I LOVE NEW YORK
EATING HOLIDAY

Orange
Canadian bacon
Slice toast with margarine (diet margarine preferred)
Coffee or tea

DAY 3: BREAKFAST   THE I LOVE NEW YORK
EATING HOLIDAY

Orange
Hot oatmeal
Low-fat milk
Coffee or tea

DAY 4: BREAKFAST

Grapefruit juice
Wheat flakes
Low-fat milk
Swiss cheese
Slice toast
Coffee or tea

DAY 5: BREAKFAST

Blend of orange and grapefruit juice
Any ready-to-eat breakfast cereal
Low-fat milk
Slice toast with margarine (diet margarine preferred)
Coffee or tea

DAY 6: BREAKFAST

Orange juice
Poached egg
Whole-wheat toast with margarine (diet margarine preferred)
Coffee or tea

DAY 7: BREAKFAST

Half grapefruit
Farina
Low-fat milk
Toast with peanut butter

LUNCH MENUS

CLIP AND PRESENT TO WAITER

DAY 1: LUNCH   THE I LOVE NEW YORK
EATING HOLIDAY

Grapefruit juice
Canned mackerel
Mixed green salad and dressing of your choice
Bread
Pickles and condiments (optional)
Any approved soft drink

DAY 2: LUNCH   THE I LOVE NEW YORK
EATING HOLIDAY

Tomato juice
Chef's salad, composed of hard-cooked eggs, lean ham, chicken,
   and dressing of your choice
Pickles and condiments (optional)
Sponge cake
Any approved soft drink

Tomato juice
Lean sliced beef
Lettuce wedges with salad dressing of your choice
Slice rye bread with margarine (diet margarine preferred)
Pickles and condiments (optional)
Angel food cake
Any approved soft drink

Tomato juice
Chopped liver
2 slices rye bread
Cucumbers and radishes
Pickles and condiments (optional)
Baked apple
Any approved soft drink

Tuna salad with dressing of your choice
Mixed raw vegetables
*Slice whole-wheat bread with margarine (diet margarine pre-
    ferred)*
Pickles and condiments (optional)
Sherbet
Any approved soft drink

DAY 6: LUNCH THE I LOVE NEW YORK
EATING HOLIDAY

Apple juice
Sliced turkey sandwich
Salad composed of raw turnip slices, pepper rings, and
   dressing of your choice
Pickles and condiments (optional)
Orange sherbet (or other fruit sherbet)
Any approved soft drink

DAY 7: LUNCH THE I LOVE NEW YORK
EATING HOLIDAY

Split-pea soup
Tossed green salad with blue-cheese dressing
Hard roll
Canned peaches (in light syrup)
Any approved soft drink

DINNER MENUS

CLIP AND PRESENT TO WAITER

DAY 1: DINNER   THE I LOVE NEW YORK
EATING HOLIDAY

Cocktail, hard liquor, beer, or wine (optional)
Chicken with noodles
Green peas
Eggplant salad
Whole-grain bread
Pickles and condiments (optional)
Melon (if not in season, any other fresh fruit)
Coffee, tea, or club soda with lemon or lime

DAY 2: DINNER   THE I LOVE NEW YORK
EATING HOLIDAY

Cocktail, hard liquor, beer, or wine (optional)
Baked fish
*Salad composed of pasta shells, cooked greens, and dressing
  of your choice*
Fresh fruit cup
Coffee, tea, or club soda with lemon or lime

DAY 3: DINNER THE I LOVE NEW YORK
EATING HOLIDAY

Cocktail, hard liquor, beer, or wine (optional)
Broiled fish
Potato salad
Cooked greens
Corn bread with margarine (diet margarine preferred)
Coffee, tea, or club soda with lemon or lime

DAY 4: DINNER THE I LOVE NEW YORK
EATING HOLIDAY

Cocktail, hard liquor, beer, or wine (optional)
Lean pork with bean sprouts
Brown rice
Spinach
Hard roll
Pickles and condiments (optional)
Pineapple cubes (fresh or packed in own juices)
Coffee, tea, or club soda with lemon or lime

DAY 5: DINNER THE I LOVE NEW YORK
EATING HOLIDAY

Cocktail, hard liquor, beer, or wine (optional)
Red beans and rice
Tomato salad with dressing of your choice
Slice bread with margarine (diet margarine preferred)
Fresh fruit cup
Coffee, tea, or club soda with lemon or lime

DAY 6: DINNER — THE I LOVE NEW YORK EATING HOLIDAY

Cocktail, hard liquor, beer, or wine (optional)
Beef stew composed of lean beef, potatoes, carrots, and onions
Tomato salad with dressing of your choice
Slice whole-wheat bread
Pickles and condiments (optional)
Fresh fruit cup
Coffee, tea, or club soda with lemon or lime

DAY 7: DINNER — THE I LOVE NEW YORK EATING HOLIDAY

Cocktail, hard liquor, beer, or wine (optional)
Roast chicken
Large baked potato
Baked squash
Cole slaw
Slice whole-wheat bread with margarine (diet margarine preferred)
Pickles and condiments (optional)
Coffee, tea, or club soda with lemon or lime

Index

IMPROVE YOUR HEALTH
WITH WARNER BOOKS